ADHD

ATTENTION DEFICIT HYPERACTIVITY DISORDER

By Dr. Rebecca Resnik, Licensed Psychologist

Published by:

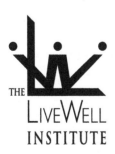

THE
LIVEWELL
INSTITUTE

www.thelivewellinstitute.com

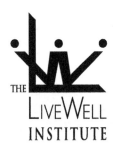

THE
LiveWell
INSTITUTE

The LiveWell Institute
PO Box 461
Herndon, VA 20172-0461 U.S.A.
www.thelivewellinstitute.com

Published by: The LiveWell Institute

Printed in the United States of America on Acid-Free Paper
10 9 8 7 6 5 4 3 2 1

ISBN: 978-0-9910592-2-5
Library of Congress Control Number: 2016955675

1. Family & Relationships / Attention Deficit Disorder (ADD-ADHD)
2. Psychology / Developmental / Child
3. Education / Special Education / Behavior and Social Disabilities

REVIEWS

"I highly recommend this book to parents and professionals who are looking to understand and support children and youth with ADHD. Dr. Resnik bases her writing on the latest research while at the same time using an accessible style with the gentle touch of a knowing mom. The quotes from parents in Dr. Resnik's practice may yield a tear but her judicious use of humor gives parents permission to laugh. I especially appreciate the 'myth busting' that will help all concerned dispel the many false beliefs surrounding ADHD. Dr. Resnik's sensible approach and advice honors both the parent and the child. I learned a lot and believe you will too."

Deborah L. Speece, Ph.D.
Associate Dean of Research and Faculty Development
Professor, Department of Counseling and Special Education
Virginia Commonwealth University

"Dr. Resnik's guide to ADHD offers compassionate and up-to-date information along with useful practical advice for families and caregivers."

Loring J. Ingraham, Ph.D.
Professor of Clinical Psychology &
Director, Professional Psychology Program
George Washington University

INTRODUCTION

If you've picked up this book, you probably have a lot of questions (and perhaps worries) running through your mind. You've probably also had a very stressful time leading up to getting your diagnosis. Every year, between 4 and 7% of parents are having this same experience – getting a diagnosis of ADHD for their child. If you think about all the families in your school, workplace, and neighborhood, that adds up to a lot of kids! You are not alone. All kinds of kids, all over the world, are coping with ADHD.

But just because ADHD diagnoses are common does not make things easy. Managing ADHD symptoms presents challenges for parent and child alike.

The good news is that because ADHD is a fairly common diagnosis, there is a lot of support out there for parents who know where to look. How do you get to be one of those savvy parents who knows how to manage ADHD? One good place to begin is with this book. This book is about learning how to manage ADHD so you, and your child, can thrive.

Here are the goals for this workbook:

1. To help you understand your child's diagnosis (and your feelings about it!)
2. To build on strengths and improve areas of need
3. To make a well-informed Action Plan

NOTE

Notes on pronouns: In order to make sure everyone can see him or herself represented in the text, I'll use 'him' and 'her,' alternating whenever possible. Unless I'm talking about issues specific to female or male parents, I use the term 'parent.' 'Parent' in this book is a generic term that refers to the greatest person or people in a child's life – the ones who give unmeasurable love and take on the daily grind of parenting work.

TABLE OF CONTENTS

PART ONE

PARENTING A CHILD WITH ADHD

CHAPTER ONE:

YOUR CHILD HAS ADHD

You've just learned something new: your child has Attention Deficit Hyperactivity Disorder.

First, take this from a psychologist: parenting DOES NOT cause ADHD. Let me repeat that – parenting DOES NOT cause ADHD. Your child's ADHD did not happen because:

- He's spoiled
- Both parents work outside the home
- You don't spank her
- You feed him non-organic food
- You let him play video games
- Kids and parents are way too soft these days

Did any of these give your kid ADHD? Of course not!

Can we please put these silly ideas to rest once and for all?

> **ADHD is a neurological difference with a strong genetic component. Kids with ADHD have a pattern of cognitive and behavioral difficulties caused by differences in how their brains function.**

This is not to underestimate the power of effective parenting, but even parents with amazing parenting skills struggle with the symptoms and behaviors of ADHD. As a former special educator turned clinical psychologist currently raising my third boy (who has ADHD), I can personally vouch for how hard it is to manage symptoms of ADHD.

Most of the basic 'good enough' parenting strategies work very well for the majority of kids. Modern parenting techniques like reasoning with kids, maintaining routines, and enforcing healthy boundaries work for about 90% of all children. If you have a kid with ADHD, you may need to learn new strategies. The 'one size fits all' approach is not going to be as useful for you. Proven parenting techniques will help your child be at his best, but parenting can't cause or cure ADHD.

Rest assured, anyone who tells you that your child has ADHD because he is spoiled or needs harsher discipline is just flat out WRONG (you might want to be a bit more diplomatic when you share that information with your mother-in-law or the equivalent 'know-it-all' in your life). Later on, I'll get into tips for how to deal with people who 'just don't get it.'

Most of the basic 'good enough' parenting strategies work very well for the majority of kids. Modern parenting techniques work for about 90% of all children. If you have a kid with ADHD, you may need to learn new strategies.

At this point, let's take a moment to laugh so we don't cry.

Here is a list of myths, ignorant statements, and just plain pigheadedness that I've heard about ADHD. And no, they aren't *really* funny, but you can laugh at other people's stupidity just this once. See which ones you have heard before:

1. French kids don't get ADHD.
2. Modern kids are just spoiled, we never had that growing up.
3. ADHD is an excuse bad parents make.
4. A good spanking would cure ADHD.
5. If he can pay attention to video games, he can't have ADHD.
6. If he doesn't have at least 6 of the DSM-5 criteria, he can't have ADHD.
7. If a child has anxiety, you can't diagnose ADHD.
8. ADHD is caused by sugar and junk food. Take that out of his diet and he'll be fine.
9. She just needs to learn better manners.
10. You know she could stop if she wanted to.
11. He's just doing it to get out of work.
12. If his academics are on grade level, he can't have a disability.
13. He'll figure it out for himself if we just get out of his way.
14. ADHD is overdiagnosed so 'big pharma' can make millions on drugs.
15. He just needs to suck it up and stop being such a baby. The world is not going to coddle him so you shouldn't either.
16. She just doesn't care about doing well.
17. ADHD is just doctors trying to make money, there's no evidence it exists.
18. He just likes failing.

MOVING FORWARD

In moving forward from the ADHD diagnosis, you may find yourself dealing with many challenges, including how to:

- Choose a school
- Advocate for the child's needs at school
- Get through homework
- Get the child ready in the morning
- Get the child settled down for bed at night
- Control impulsive behavior
- Help the child make and keep friends
- Keep the child motivated
- Improve the child's personal organization
- Cope with emotional 'ups and downs' (your child's *and* yours)
- Help the child get along with siblings

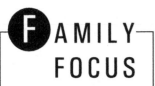

FAMILY FOCUS

"I wish I had known how impaired her attention and memory were years ago. My wife and I have been reprimanding her and even punishing her for things that we now know she couldn't control."

4

The good news is that once you get an action plan in place, you can pull together a team to help. Families who try to 'go it alone' often face years of largely unnecessary stress and frustration. Later in this workbook we'll go over how to create this plan. But right now, we're at the beginning: your child has just been diagnosed with ADHD.

There are serious costs to *not* getting your child diagnosed or having your child misdiagnosed:

- Individuals with ADHD are more likely to suffer from anxiety or depression.

- They are at higher risk for failing to achieve their potential at school, at work, and in relationships.

- Research has shown that people with ADHD are more likely to engage in high-risk behavior that may result in situations like getting into a car accident or using illicit substances.

If left undiagnosed and untreated, ADHD can cause a lot of emotional distress. Children with ADHD face years of 'not measuring up' and wondering what is wrong with them. This is especially true in elementary school, where the key to success is being able to sit still, pay attention, and get your work done with minimal help. Kids with ADHD have to work so much harder to do all of these things. They are often exhausted and discouraged by fourth grade. Over time, they become more aware of their differences as they watch their friends succeed with far less effort.

THE DIFFERENCE BETWEEN A LABEL AND A DIAGNOSIS

You DON'T want your child labeled. However, there is a critical difference between a label and a diagnosis. In my practice, I have seen many kids who went without help for their ADHD because somebody was afraid of a getting a label.

A LABEL

People love labels because they are easy – they help us make sense of our world by putting people into categories. That's just how our brains work. We categorize things so we don't have to work as hard to understand them. But labels lock us into roles.

- ✔ Labels describe what *other people* see when they look at us
- ✔ Labels are not the truth
- ✔ Labels don't promote understanding, they create distance
- ✔ Labels don't help with problem solving, in fact, they shut it down

So when a parent (usually a father) tells me he doesn't want his kid labeled, I tell him he's absolutely right. That said, I am not the one who is going to label his kid. The people who are going to do it are the teachers, coaches, other parents, relatives and all the people out there who are making judgments based on what they see.

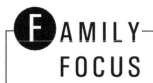

FAMILY FOCUS

"We took the kids over to my sister's house for a play date with the cousins. The very first thing my sister did was take Ryan over to a corner and show him the time out chair."

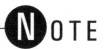

NOTE

Labels pop up like mushrooms – they grow in the dark. It is your job as a parent to shed light on your child's struggles so that labels will fade in the light of understanding.

A DIAGNOSIS

A diagnosis communicates information about a condition.
It provides a framework for understanding what is happening. We are used to having our kids diagnosed with medical issues – strep throat, ear infections, etc. Diagnosis of ADHD is different because there's no quick and easy test that gives an absolute answer, and diagnostic criteria are changing as the field advances.

Diagnosis of a psychiatric or cognitive disability means that there is a particular set of neurological differences causing a pattern of observable symptoms and/or behaviors. This means that the person's brain is functioning differently from that of same-aged peers, and thus, her behavior or functioning differ too. A thorough diagnosis gives meaning to behavioral observations.

The diagnosis communicates that there is a pattern of differences
that is largely consistent across individuals with ADHD.

At this time it is easier, and more useful, to observe behavior than it is to observe brain function (the scientific community is still trying to understand exactly what brain differences underlie specific deficits associated with ADHD).

Most importantly, a diagnosis promotes problem solving.
A diagnosis of ADHD points us towards interventions that will work, including treatments, therapies and accommodations. Once you have that diagnosis, your job as a parent is twofold.

 First: Help the people in your child's life understand her diagnosis accurately.

Second: Help people see beyond the diagnosis so they can understand your child as a unique individual and avoid using labels.

A diagnosis of ADHD points us towards interventions that will work, including treatments, therapies and accommodations.

CHAPTER TWO:

THE DIAGNOSIS

WHO STARTS THE PROCESS?

Here's a list of the professionals who can (and should!) point out symptoms of concern to you. However, the professionals on this list cannot diagnose ADHD by themselves:

- Speech Language Pathologists
- Occupational and Physical Therapists
- Tutors, Teachers
- School Administrators
- Guidance Counselors
- Dieticians
- Daycare Providers

YOUR CRITICAL ROLE AS A PARENT

A diagnosis of ADHD is not like strep throat, where the doctor does a test and gives you a diagnosis. ADHD has to be diagnosed through careful observation of behavior.

For starters, keep in mind that not all children who have trouble controlling their attention or impulses have ADHD, and not all kids with ADHD have trouble paying attention!

Because it is so complicated, ADHD is a 'diagnosis of exclusion.' Making the diagnosis means that there can be **no other better explanation** for the child's symptoms. On a practical level, that means checking for other conditions that can mimic ADHD (and there are a bunch).

A diagnosis of ADHD is not like strep throat, where the doctor does a test and gives you a diagnosis. ADHD has to be diagnosed through careful observation of behavior.

Physical conditions can mimic (and co-exist with) ADHD. The more conditions you have circled in Exercise #1, the more you need to get additional information to be confident that your child's diagnosis is accurate.

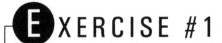

EXERCISE #1

HELP YOUR DOCTOR RULE OUT PHYSICAL DISORDERS

Physical conditions can mimic (and co-exist with) ADHD. Below, circle any that might apply to your child. The more you have circled, the more you need to get additional information to be confident that your child's diagnosis is accurate.

- Sleep disorder (including: apnea/restricted airway, night terrors, trouble falling or staying asleep)

- Thyroid problems

- Developmental delays

- Anemia

- Blood sugar regulation problems

- Hearing impairment

- Visual impairment

- Sleep deprivation (especially among teenagers getting less than 8 hours per night)

- Use of illicit substances (especially marijuana)

- Neurological impairments (e.g. seizure disorder)

- High functioning Autism Spectrum Disorder

- Sensory hyposensitivities or hypersensitivities (under- or over-reacting to sensory input)

- Allergies/reactions to particular foods

- Exposure to lead

Most of these will be excluded as part of a thorough annual physical. If you are worried about any items noted here, don't wait for your doctor to raise the issue. Take this list with you so you don't forget anything.

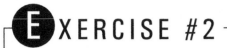

EXERCISE #2

ASK YOUR DOCTOR ABOUT MENTAL HEALTH AND COGNITIVE PROBLEMS THAT CAN MIMIC ADHD

Below are psychological and cognitive conditions that can mimic ADHD. Do not expect your pediatrician to spot these in a routine physical! Children behave differently when they're at the doctors'. You're the only one who can tell your doctor what your child is really like.

- Anxiety

- Unusual or extreme fears

- Problems making and keeping friends

- Uncooperative behavior at home or school

- Hyperactivity/impulsivity

- High levels of stress (may include grief or life transitions)

- History of trauma

- Learning difficulties or disabilities

- Depression (may look like irritability or anger management problems)

- Trouble understanding language

- Trouble using language or communicating with others

- Abuse or maltreatment (including bullying)

- Obsessions and compulsions

- Autism Spectrum Disorder

Again, your doctor is counting on you to bring up any behavior or learning concerns you have. Be ready to bring them up clearly and efficiently (remember, your doctor has about 15 minutes!). Writing out your concerns ahead of time will make sure you get to ask about them all.

Psychological and cognitive conditions listed in Exercise #2 can mimic ADHD. Do not expect your pediatrician to spot these in a routine physical!

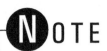

NOTE

Physicians have terrific training in diagnosing and treating medical problems. Not all have as in-depth knowledge about mental health. Sometimes their knowledge is out of date. For example, I still hear professionals tell parents things like, "well, if he can pay attention to video games it can't be ADHD." Or, "if the child is anxious than it can't be ADHD." It is important to recognize what is within your physician's area of expertise, and to know when to seek other experts.

WORKING WITH YOUR CHILD'S DOCTOR

Tip 1. Ask questions.

As a parent, see it as your role to ask questions. You may not be comfortable asking or you may not feel that your doctor welcomes questions (if needed, schedule a separate appointment so you can talk just about you concerns). The most important thing is getting an accurate diagnosis, and you are a critical part of that process, so voice your concerns! If you are worried about being brushed aside (especially true for mothers or parents who have trouble speaking English), bring a relative or friend who can speak for you. If your doctor does not take you seriously, hopefully there are other doctors nearby who will.

Tip 2. Don't expect your doctor to be a mind reader.

Do you believe your doctor can read your mind? No, of course not. Don't make the mistake of thinking that if the doctor does not see something that concerns you, that everything is fine! Remember, your pediatrician only has about 15 minutes to do a full examination. He has a long checklist of things to look at and think about in that time. In such a brief time, your doctor is unlikely to see symptoms of many childhood problems – she's working as fast as she can to do the physical. The doctor depends on you to be clear and explicit about your concerns.

Tip 3. Trust your instincts.

As parents, we often know when something is off. In my professional life, I have heard of many families who were told to 'wait and see' or who had their concerns shrugged off by professionals. If nothing was wrong, that's great – the clinician saved the family a lot of heartache (and money!). But if there is something amiss, intervening early is critical. Small problems are easier to fix (and again, cheaper to fix) than big problems. If you have concerns, don't stop with one professional. Get more opinions and find someone with the expertise you need.

ONCE OTHER CONDITIONS HAVE BEEN EXCLUDED, HOW IS ADHD DIAGNOSED?

Once other conditions are ruled out, diagnosing ADHD becomes a process of systematic observation. Remember, since ADHD is a diagnosis of exclusion, one type of information is not enough to figure out what is behind the symptoms and behaviors. And because ADHD symptoms and behaviors occur in specific settings, the clinician needs to understand how the child is doing at home, school, community, and in social relationships.

HERE ARE WAYS CLINICIANS GATHER INFORMATION TO HELP THEM DIAGNOSE ADHD:

- Observing the child in the office
- Clinical Interview (with the parents and child)
- Observation of the child at home or school
- Parent report of symptoms
- Behavioral Rating Scales (questionnaires for parents and teachers that ask about symptoms and behaviors associated with ADHD, such as the Vanderbilt, BRIEF, Conners or CEFI)
- Psychological Testing (performance-based measures that ask the child to solve problems and compare him to same-aged peers, such as IQ tests and continuous performance tests)
- Neurological examination

Once the professional collects information about the child, she needs to determine if the child's profile of symptoms and behaviors matches the diagnostic criteria for ADHD. Let's look at two ways information can be collected:

- Behavioral Diagnostic Roadmaps
- Neuropsychological Testing

BEHAVIORAL DIAGNOSTIC ROADMAPS_____

DSM-5 AND ICD-10: TWO BEHAVIORAL ROADMAPS USED TO DIAGNOSE ADHD

Historically, ADHD has been diagnosed based on observations of the child's behavior. Making the diagnosis meant checking for at least six of the symptoms from the diagnostic criteria defined in the *Diagnostic and Statistical Manual of the American Psychiatric Association* (DSM, now in its fifth edition, DSM-5). Practitioners across the world could also use the World Health Organization's *International Classification of Diseases* (these ICD-10 'disease' codes are the same ones you see on your insurance bills under diagnosis).

ICD refers to ADHD as a behavior disorder impacting inattention, hyperactivity, and impulsivity.
The problems have to be inappropriate for the child's age (e.g. needing to run around more than most 8-year-old boys). Both DSM and ICD require that symptoms begin in childhood. The American Academy of Pediatrics recently took the position that ADHD can be diagnosed in children as young as four years old. ADHD symptoms also have to be present across settings, such as home, school, and in the community according to DSM and ICD.

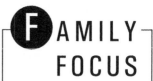

FAMILY FOCUS

"Our daughter had everybody fooled. The school team told us that everything was fine, that she was just not very smart and that she was doing about what we could expect. This did not hit us right at all. She was basically phoning it in at school, doing the minimum to keep a low profile. We just didn't believe that lowering our expectations was the right choice, so we decided to find out for ourselves. The testing showed that she was actually highly gifted and very anxious. Whenever she got bored or nervous, she'd start daydreaming. I think she must have spent most of the day zoned out for years. She just played the part of the perfect, quiet girl."

Many clinicians in mental health use the DSM-5, so you need to familiarize yourself with what it says.

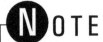 **N**OTE

Not everyone agrees that the DSM is the ultimate authority on diagnosis. In fact, the International Classification of Disease diagnostic system (ICD-1) is most used worldwide. It is the position of the American Psychological Association that psychologists may use either ICD or DSM. That said, many clinicians in mental health use the DSM-5, so you need to familiarize yourself with what it says.

The DSM-5 includes three types of ADHD:
• Inattentive
• Hyperactive-Impulsive
• Combined Type (symptoms from both 'menus' are present)

*For **Inattentive Type ADHD** (for children through age 17), the DSM requires 6 of the following symptoms:*

• Fails to give close attention to details or makes careless mistakes
• Has difficulty sustaining attention
• Does not appear to listen
• Struggles to follow-through on instructions
• Has difficulty with organization
• Avoids or dislikes tasks requiring a lot of thinking
• Loses things
• Is easily distracted
• Is forgetful in daily activities

*For **Hyperactive-Impulsive Type** (for children through age 17), the DSM requires 6 of the following symptoms:*

• Fidgets with hands or feet, or squirms in chair
• Has difficulty remaining seated
• Runs about or climbs excessively (in children) (Feelings of restlessness in adults)
• Difficulty engaging in activities quietly
• Acts as if driven by a motor (adults will experience restlessness)
• Talks excessively. Blurts out answers before questions have been completed
• Difficulty waiting or taking turns
• Interrupts or intrudes upon others

The DSM-5 is more specific than ICD.

DSM-5 lists behaviors. This is helpful if your child happens to exhibit these behaviors and everyone filling out the rating scales agrees (this happens far less frequently than you might think!). Remember that not every child with a significant attentional control issue will fit neatly into a checklist-based system. Children who are gifted or whose symptoms are more subtle (like many girls) may be under-identified or misdiagnosed. According to the DSM authors, if a child has six (or an adult has five) items on the DSM checklist, she meets diagnostic criteria.

What behaviors do *you* see?

A good practice is for you to run through the same checklist of behaviors that clinicians might use to diagnose your child.

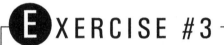

EXERCISE #3

WHAT BEHAVIORS DO YOU SEE?

Mark any and all of these behaviors that apply to your child. As you work through the exercise, you may find that you, too, meet the diagnostic criteria for ADHD. Since ADHD runs in families many parents discover they had the same problems as children, and that those problems may not have gone away.

For **Inattentive Type ADHD**, the DSM requires 6 of the following symptoms:

_____ Fails to give close attention to details or makes careless mistakes
___/__ Has difficulty sustaining attention
___/__ Does not appear to listen
_____ Struggles to follow-through on instructions
___/__ Has difficulty with organization
_____ Avoids or dislikes tasks requiring a lot of thinking
_____ Loses things
_____ Is easily distracted
_____ Is forgetful in daily activities

For **Hyperactive-Impulsive Type**, the DSM identifies the following symptoms:

___/ Fidgets with hands or feet, or squirms in chair
___/ Has difficulty remaining seated
___/ Runs about or climbs excessively
___/ Difficulty engaging in activities quietly
___/ Acts as if driven by a motor
___/ Talks excessively. Blurts out answers before questions have been completed
___/ Difficulty waiting or taking turns
___/ Interrupts or intrudes upon others

You may find that you, too, meet the diagnostic criteria for ADHD. Since ADHD runs in families many parents discover they had the same problems as children, and that those problems may not have gone away.

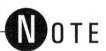

NOTE

The problem with relying exclusively on behavior-based systems and subjective raters is not that ADHD gets overdiagnosed, but that it is *misdiagnosed*. Another problem with the behavior-based system is that too many kids get 'lumped' into the ADHD diagnostic category.

Difficulty focusing and sustaining attention is a feature of many pediatric psychiatric and cognitive disorders, not just ADHD. Researchers have argued that this emphasis on overt behaviors in diagnosis is why our treatments don't work as well for all children as we would expect.

Notice how these criteria are based entirely on *behavior*?
You can see that the behaviors in the second set – those related to hyperactivity, are much easier for people to notice! A child who is up out of his seat or leaping off the top of the monkey bars at recess attracts attention. The child who daydreams all day about Harry Potter or Minecraft is much harder to spot (especially if that child is bright enough to keep up in spite of the distractibility). Hence girls, who tend to have more inattentive symptoms, are often not diagnosed until they are far older than boys.

There's a lot of subjectivity in observing behaviors.
Whereas one teacher might say that a child 'talks excessively,' the parent might not. The parent might not notice any problem with paying attention at home, while the teacher might see a child who cannot finish any classwork. What one observer may consider highly unusual might not phase someone else.

There are gender issues to consider as well.
A high activity level in a boy 'stands-out' less than that same energy level in a girl. We also know that boys and girls typically present different sets of symptoms. Boys tend to show more disruptive behaviors. Girls can have severe attention control issues that go unnoticed if they are quiet.

DON'T CLOUD THE DIAGNOSIS

Every person filling out the rating scale has his or her own bias. Sometimes, raters have a deliberate agenda in mind. For example, some parents and teachers are invested in 'getting a child help.' They may fill out the rating scale to show as many problems as possible. Other raters want to 'prove' that there is nothing wrong with their child. They may endorse few items or minimize the severity.

It is important not to let advocating for the child's needs cloud the diagnostic picture – after all, accurate diagnosis is the bedrock of effective treatment.

Hidden sources of bias matter.

Research has shown that more mothers than fathers tend to rate children as having problems. Research has also shown that African American and Hispanic/Latino children are often judged differently by raters. African American children are more likely to be referred for special education services. They are also likely to be disciplined and suspended more frequently than Caucasian children. Behavior of African American children is often perceived to be more problematic than *the same* behaviors exhibited by Caucasian children. While parents and professionals need to be mindful of our own hidden biases, we should not over-correct to the extent that we fail to identify children with disabilities (worst case scenario is labeling a child as 'bad' without trying to understand her behavior).

WHAT HAPPENS WHEN THERE'S DISAGREEMENT ON THE DIAGNOSIS?

What do you do when one set of results shows the child meets diagnostic criteria while other results do not?

For example, research shows that mothers tend to report more ADHD symptoms than fathers. So if the mother's ratings are positive for ADHD, and the fathers are not, what is the professional to do?

Teachers also often have different opinions, particularly once the child is in middle and high school. These teachers do not spend the same amount of time with a child as an elementary school teacher. The differences in the demands of each class can bring forth very different behaviors in a child (e.g. Jay, who loves science but hates English, might be rated by the science teacher as not disabled, but an hour later in the day he's causing major disruptions in English class).

The key to making an accurate diagnosis of ADHD is to get *multiple* sources of data. In 2013, Dr. Tom Insel, Director of the National Institute of Mental Health, was among those who called for psychological and cognitive disorders to be diagnosed based on what is happening in people's brains, not just their behavior.

This makes sense because – as we've seen earlier – relying solely on people's subjective observations can be problematic. This is true whether we are thinking of the psychiatrist who reaches a diagnosis using an interview, or parents and teachers completing behavioral rating scales.

Plus, behavior-based diagnoses are limited when it comes to predicting what interventions will work.

African American children are more likely to be referred for special education services. They are also likely to be disciplined and suspended more frequently than Caucasian children.

The key to making an accurate diagnosis of ADHD is to get multiple sources of data.

*Neuropsychological testing assesses all the major areas of cognitive functioning with the goal of understanding how your child's brain works. **It gives you a broad profile of his strengths and weaknesses so you can focus your interventions.***

NEUROPSYCHOLOGICAL TESTING _____

THE NEW BEST PRACTICE: 'BRAIN-BASED' VS. BEHAVIOR-BASED DIAGNOSIS

A diagnosis should always include gathering data, preferably multiple sources of information. Among these are **performance-based measures**, or what we refer to as psychological (or neuropsychological) testing. The term 'neuropsychological' means that the clinician is trying to understand your child in terms of what we know about brain function.

Psychological tests allow for structured observation of how well the child's brain solves different kinds of problems.
This helps us understand WHY behaviors are happening. For example, if we test and find that a child has a very slow *processing speed*, that helps us understand why it takes so long for her to get her work done. If we test a child and find that he has trouble *recalling information* for more than a few minutes, that helps us understand why he can't follow multistep directions.

Neuropsychological testing offers us a much richer basis for making an ADHD diagnosis and planning interventions.

WHY GET MORE EXTENSIVE TESTING?

Neuropsychological testing can be expensive (if you go with a private practice) or time consuming (if you end up on a hospital's wait list). So why do it?

Remember that ADHD is a diagnosis of exclusion. That means that the diagnosing clinician has to rule out other possible conditions. ADHD is also a disorder that tends to appear with other disorders, including learning difficulties, anxiety, and depression. Neuropsychological testing assesses all the major areas of cognitive functioning with the goal of understanding how your child's brain works. **It gives you a broad profile of his strengths and weaknesses so you can focus your interventions.**

GOOD REASONS FOR PURSUING NEUROPSYCHOLOGICAL TESTING INCLUDE:

- You are not sure the diagnosis is correct
- Your current interventions are not making things better
- You need a deeper understanding of your child's strengths and weaknesses
- Your child is complex – other factors may be in play, such as giftedness, anxiety, learning disabilities, speech/language delays, or behavior difficulties
- Your child has another condition that could be creating attentional control problems (e.g. epilepsy, autism spectrum disorder, a genetic difference, thyroid problems etc.)

WHEN SHOULD I HAVE MY CHILD TESTED?

There are many opinions. In my experience, getting testing earlier saves a lot of stress, frustration, and even money. Waiting until things reach a crisis – or until your child has been struggling for years – makes problems bigger and harder to fix. Once a child has begun to hate school or think she is stupid or bad, it is particularly hard to help her feel hope again. Likewise, it is easier to fix a small lag in achievement than to get a child caught up after he is well behind his peers, particularly in the early years of elementary school. Unaddressed, ADHD can create a lot of damage that you won't see until it becomes a BIG problem that costs considerable time and money to fix.

But specifically, when should a child be tested?

There is no 'right' time that works for all children, though sooner is generally better. Here are common times to get testing:

- After you have that first talk with the pediatrician about her symptoms and behaviors
- When a professional in the child's life (someone you trust) recommends it
- Before the first eligibility meeting at school, or before the IEP/504 Plan is written
- In preparation for major school changes, such as before 3rd, 6th, or 9th grades
- When your child is preparing to take 'high stakes' standardized tests in high school (remember, you need to get the testing done at least 3 months before to make sure you have time to complete the accommodations application process! So start calling psychologists about 6 months before you want your child to take standardized tests!)

Unaddressed, ADHD can create a lot of damage that you won't see until it becomes a BIG problem that costs considerable time and money to fix.

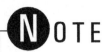

N O T E

The testing done in the public school system can be right for many children. But if the interventions put in place after that testing aren't working, it's a sign that more extensive testing could be needed to support your child's needs and progress.

If a child is not ___well below___ *grade level, some educators will say that there is no 'educational impact.' This is not true. Educational impact is not just achieving below grade level.*

Keep in mind that many school professionals still have a 'wait to fail' mentality.

They may tell you there is no reason to test your child. In fact, if a child is not *well below* grade level, some educators will say that there is no 'educational impact.' This is not true. Educational impact is not just achieving below grade level (more on this later). Such 'old school' professionals may use big words to make you feel small. They may imply that you are just a 'helicopter parent' or an overanxious mom (I never hear the term overanxious dad!). If you have good reason to believe that something is wrong, don't accept this answer.

Also, some school professionals will tell you that they cannot test a child of a certain age...

or that they have to try Response to Intervention (RTI) before your child can be tested. Neither of these is true. Children of all ages (even infants!) can be tested to gauge their development. RTI interventions do not prevent testing. A child can be tested while receiving *any level* of RTI services. It may make sense to wait for a bit, to see if the RTI interventions help (for example, meeting with a reading specialist for intensive help with decoding). Some kids will get what they need from RTI. That said, if your child is not making expected progress, it is ok at any point to request testing or get an outside evaluation.

What does neuropsychological testing involve? Comprehensive neuropsychological testing includes formal assessment of the following:

- Intelligence
- Expressive and receptive language
- Information processing
- Executive functioning
- Memory
- Visual spatial processing
- Developmental history
- Behavior
- Daily living skills

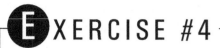

EXERCISE #4

DOES YOUR CHILD NEED A COMPREHENSIVE OR NEUROPSYCHOLOGICAL EVALUATION?

TAKE THIS QUICK QUIZ:

1. Does the diagnosis of ADHD address all the problem symptoms/ behaviors?

2. Do you have additional concerns about your child's mood, behavior, or social life?

3. Is your child making appropriate academic progress at school?

4. If not, are you getting the right help at school so your child can make progress?

5. Is medication working well enough that you can say it is making life better?

6. Are behavioral interventions at home and school working?

7. Is your life, and your child's life getting better?

If you answered 'no' or thought 'not really' to more than one of these questions, you need more information. Neuropsychological testing can help you understand more about what is happening with your child. Once you understand *why* things are not getting better, you can move forward with a customized, data-based plan.

Some school professionals will tell you that they cannot test a child of a certain age, or that they have to try Response to Intervention (RTI) before your child can be tested. Neither of these is true.

Another way to evaluate how your child has been diagnosed is to look at who did the diagnosis. Professionals and clinicians in different specialties were trained to approach diagnosing ADHD differently. By looking at the type of professional(s) involved, you gain insights into the scope of information – behavioral and testing-wise – that was used to determine your child's diagnosis.

Professionals and clinicians in different specialties were trained to approach diagnosing ADHD differently. By looking at the type of professional(s) involved, you gain insights into the scope of information – behavioral and testing-wise – that was used to determine your child's diagnosis.

EXERCISE #5

WHO DIAGNOSED YOUR CHILD?

Check off who helped to diagnose your child. Note the types of information they used:

❑ **Physician:** parent report of symptoms, behavioral rating scales (the American Academy of Pediatrics encourages physicians to use behavior rating scales but not all do. Typically, medical doctors use the Vanderbilt scales)

❑ **Psychiatrist:** clinical interview with parent and child, behavior rating scales

❑ **Neurologist:** neurological exam, clinical interview with parent and child, behavior rating scales

❑ **Master's Level Therapist (Counselor, Social Worker):** clinical interview with parent and child, behavior rating scales, possibly observation

❑ **School Psychologist:** IQ test, classroom observation/Functional Behavioral Analysis (a structured observation where data are collected about behavior), and behavioral rating scales

❑ **Clinical Psychologist:** clinical interview with parent and child, performance-based psychological tests, behavioral rating scales (may include formal observation outside of the office)

❑ **Neuropsychologist:** clinical interview with parent and child, performance-based psychological tests, behavioral rating scales (may include formal observation outside of the office)

Some rating scales like the Vanderbilt are primarily for screening. Screening measures are often short lists of symptoms and behaviors. They are not as good at ruling out other things that could be mimicking ADHD.

Other more in-depth rating scales are more useful in making a diagnosis. Rating scales are lists of questions asking about your child's symptoms and behaviors. Your responses are scored. The scores compare your child to same-aged, same-gender peers. Tools such as the Conners Rating Scales, Behavior Rating Inventory of Executive Functioning, Comprehensive Executive Functioning Inventory, Child Behavior Checklist, and Behavior Assessment Scale for Children are well-regarded behavior rating scales used in diagnosis.

CHAPTER THREE:

BENCHMARKING AND WHAT TO EXPECT

An ADHD diagnosis confirms that your child is 'different' from his typical peers. But *how* is he different? And what unique strengths can serve him in dealing with his ADHD?

The first step is to understand what 'normal' development looks like in terms of the tasks that kids can typically be expected to manage within each age group. You may find that your child is not really all that different from his peers in quite a few areas.

TYPICAL DEVELOPMENTAL MILESTONES _____

PRESCHOOL

- Run simple errands (i.e. "put your plate and cup in the trash can")
- Perform simple chores and self-help tasks with reminders (i.e. "put on your shoes, hang up your coat")
- Inhibit behaviors: don't touch a hot stove, don't run into the street, don't snatch a toy from another child, don't hit, don't bite, etc.
- Tolerate activities that require focus and self-control for short periods of time (i.e. circle time, story time)

What may be different with ADHD:
Little kids with ADHD have trouble inhibiting impulses. They may be the kids at the play group who bite or hit. They may be the ones who don't notice they have to urinate until it is an emergency, and frequently come home with wet pants. Little kids with ADHD have trouble sitting still during circle time or work time. They may be too loud or too wild for the situation. They may play too roughly. They may find it very difficult to settle down for a nap, and may spend nap time kicking or rolling around instead of sleeping.

The first step is to understand what 'normal' development looks like in terms of the tasks that kids can typically be expected to manage within each age group.

Children with ADHD usually do not have significant academic problems through second grade unless there is a co-occurring learning disability.

KINDERGARTEN – GRADE 2

- Bring papers to and from school
- Complete homework/schoolwork assignments (20 minutes maximum)
- Inhibit behaviors: follow safety rules, don't use 'potty talk' or foul language, raise hand before speaking in class, keep hands to self
- Begin to consider the feelings of others before acting

What may be different with ADHD:
Kindergarten is usually a pretty good year for kids with ADHD, but when parents look back, they can often see the seeds of the disorder starting to sprout. First grade is a year of introducing new skills and concepts. Many tasks are quick and single step. Second grade is a consolidation year, where skills are expanded and fluency is developed. Children with ADHD usually do not have significant academic problems through second grade unless there is a co-occurring learning disability. What parents usually hear is reports of being off task and too impulsive. Teachers may express concerns about academics, but often encourage parents to 'wait and see.'

GRADES 3 – 5

- Perform chores that take 15-30 minutes long (cleaning up his/her room or toys)
- Keep track of belongings when away from home
- Complete homework assignments (work for 30 minutes or more)
- Keep track of changing daily schedule (different activities after school)

Social expectations change a lot in third to fifth grade too. Children are expected to be more considerate of each other and of adults. Meltdowns are now unusual (and very unwelcome events). Kids this age can usually take part in a lot of activities. They are generally calm and focused enough to tolerate learning a lot of new things like musical instruments or how to play team sports.

Psychologists see a lot of children with ADHD when they hit third grade ... this is when we most often hear about our kids saying they no longer like school.

What may be different with ADHD:
Psychologists see a lot of children with ADHD when they hit third grade. Third grade is an 'application year.' This means that kids are expected to have developed automaticity (working with little effort, skills like reading are 'automatic') and fluency (speed, efficiency). This is the year that tasks become longer and more detailed. If you are shaky or too slow with any of your basic foundational skills, this is where your 'castle on the sand' starts to topple. Reading changes from 'learning to read' to 'reading to learn.' Extended writing is also part of the day. Children go from writing a few sentences to writing reports and paragraphs. All of the academic tasks shift over to tasks requiring sustained attention to detail. This is often the downfall of many of our kids with ADHD. It is also when we most often hear about our kids saying they no longer like school.

At this age, kids are expected to be good sports when they lose. Boys are expected to be less physical. For girls, the social scene changes to include complex and subtle relationships. Girls typically have rapidly maturing verbal skills at this age. They adeptly use sarcasm, figurative language, and gossip to communicate amongst themselves. Subtle nonverbal behaviors such as eye rolling or a toss of the hair can speak volumes. Inattentive girls who miss these cues may find themselves confused or locked out of the 'in-crowd.'

Hierarchies among girls and boys emerge. Bullying, exclusion or shunning often 'ramps up' at this age, particularly among girls. This also the era when the 'popular' group begins to take shape. Children begin to compare themselves unfavorably to these popular kids, and may be willing to do almost anything to be accepted by them. Kids with impulse control problems may make unwise choices to be accepted (e.g. clowning around in class, using inappropriate humor, taking dares).

GRADES 6 – 8

- Use system for organizing schoolwork; including assignment book, notebooks, etc.
- Follow complex school schedule involving changing teachers and changing schedules
- Plan and carry out long-term projects, including tasks to be accomplished and reasonable timelines to follow; may require planning multiple large projects simultaneously
- Navigate the complicated, ever-changing world of peer relationships
- Cope with the physical changes of puberty and manage hygiene
- Tolerate the changing relationship with parents without serious behavior problems

The organizational demands escalate sharply, leaving kids who relied on the structure of elementary school to 'keep it together' scrambling.

This is universally recognized as a tough time for kids, but middle school has a lot of wonderful things about it too. Children are starting to learn to think in new and exciting ways. They are ready to take on more responsibility. They are typically ready for new adventures like sleep away camp or going to the movies by themselves.

Middle school can be a high-stress time academically. The organizational demands escalate sharply, leaving kids who relied on the structure of elementary school to 'keep it together' scrambling. Expectations such as coming to every class prepared can be overwhelming. Kids are supposed to have their elementary school foundational skills mastered and be fluent in preparation for higher order thinking tasks (reading novels, pre-algebra). They will now have more regular tests and quizzes that will count towards letter grades.

FAMILY FOCUS

"When she was in kindergarten she got invited to lots of birthday parties, because of course, everyone invited everyone. As the years have gone on, I'm grateful if she gets one a year. She's so lonely, but her behavior makes the other kids avoid her. I get why they don't invite her, but God it hurts."

Middle schoolers also need to manage changing relationships between peers, siblings and parents. We often hear the misconception that teenagers are 'horrible' or that it is normal for them to hate their parents. This is just not so! Research shows that most teens do not have behavior problems or significant strife. Yes, there are bumps along the way, and yes, you may see unattractive behaviors (eye rolling, sarcasm, wearing strange clothes). Though teens can be difficult to live with sometimes, they are also really interesting people. They have boundless energy, fresh new ideas, and they get very passionate about things they care about.

What may be different with ADHD:

The self-absorption of early adolescence is a normal part of development. Their brains are going through a major structural overhaul. The brain is literally reconstructing itself to prepare for adulthood. While self-absorption is expected, it should lead to a greater capacity for self-awareness. Teens with ADHD will stand out as immature. They lack age-appropriate capacity for self-reflection. They continue to need more adult support than expected from their parents and teachers.

Young teens with ADHD often struggle with impulsivity, and often make foolish mistakes even though they know better. Teens with ADHD are more likely to struggle with anxiety and depression, and to have more trouble managing daily stress. Unfortunately, this puts them at higher risk for turning to problematic behaviors (drinking, smoking, promiscuity, shoplifting, cutting, etc.). You might think these problems are not issues until high school. The research shows otherwise – that many of these problematic behaviors actually begin in middle school. What your child does during these critical years will shape who they become. If you see behavior problems budding, it is critical to act fast and get professional help!

But not all young teens with ADHD are impulsive. For many, executive functioning problems (organization, time management, task completion) become more severe problems than ever. Teens with ADHD may struggle more with academics than they did in elementary school. Problems like poor time management or forgetting to turn in homework assignments can become major headaches for the teen and his parents. Since teens are 'programmed' to want to be more independent, they may resist accepting the help they desperately need.

HIGH SCHOOL

- Manage schoolwork effectively on a day to day basis, including completing and handing in assignments on time, studying for tests, creating and following timelines for long term projects and making adjustments in effort, and quality of work in response to feedback from teachers and others (i.e. grades on tests, papers)
- Establish and refine a long term goal and make plans for meeting that goal
- Maintain positive relationships with parents and teachers
- Learn to drive or to use public transportation
- Learn to be safe in the community without adult supervision
- Begin to manage their own money
- Have a first job (typically babysitting, dog walking or lawn mowing)

As high school students grow older, their maturing frontal lobe allows for more control over their attention, executive functioning and emotional life. The emotional drama of the early teen years typically settles down, and teens begin to take on more adult responsibilities. They also gain more freedoms very rapidly. Teens are generally expected to manage their own school work, homework and classwork. Most will have a job, work study, or internship on top of school work. Teachers are not as able to stay on top of a student to make sure he follows through, so many kids 'fall through the cracks.' Freshman year is particularly difficult for boys.

What may be different with ADHD:
As previously stated, it is normal for a teen to make mistakes or even be hard to tolerate sometimes. Remember, the brain is undergoing a big developmental reboot that will not be done until age 25. Each teen will mature at his or her own pace. Keep in mind – it is NOT normal to have constant arguing, use of illicit substances, flaunting of family rules, aggressiveness/self-harming behavior, or refusal to make an effort at school.

These behaviors are red flags that the parent and school must take action, not sit back and wait. Behaviors that put your child (or anyone else) at risk, damage property, or break the law must not be tolerated. Just because a teen has ADHD does not make these behaviors acceptable.

Teens with ADHD may look physically mature, but they are emotionally immature. Their bodies look like adults, but their minds can function much more like that of a child. This puts them at risk for making unwise choices. They may be more likely to make a poor choice such as accepting a ride from a stranger, trying drugs, doing a dangerous stunt to impress friends, or shoplifting. Of course not all teens with ADHD are going to engage in these behaviors, but high levels of impulsivity combined with low self-esteem raise the risk. Keep in mind that kids with ADHD who misbehave may not be malicious, and they may be surprised that other people get upset. They

It is NOT normal to have constant arguing, use of illicit substances, flaunting of family rules, aggressiveness/ self-harming behavior, or refusal to make an effort at school.

Older teens with ADHD are at higher risk for emotional problems, including anxiety and depression.

most often act without thinking. All of us are most vulnerable to making foolish choices when we feel bad when we feel frustrated, disrespected, threatened, overlooked or undervalued. This does not excuse the behavior, but helps us understand how we can change it.

Teens with ADHD need a higher level of support at school during these years. They may also resist it. This resistance is developmentally appropriate – part of the struggle for independence, but it can make it harder to help a teen who does not recognize that she NEEDS help! Teens are less likely to accept help and guidance from parents than they are from trusted adults outside the family. Parents may need to get a team of caring adults involved.

Supports such as 504 Plans (more on this later), tutors or coaches can make all the difference. Teens with ADHD typically have a hard time managing the organizational demands of school. They may not turn in homework. They have weak time management skills. They may lose things and are often unprepared for class or sports. Teens with ADHD tend to be passive in their studying, and use ineffective techniques. They may also make a habit of procrastinating, particularly if they know a parent will bail them out! Don't let your teen lock you into this pattern – it may feel good to be able to 'save the day' but for routine responsibilities you need to resist the urge to do it for them. Doing nothing is far harder than 'saving the day.'

Older teens with ADHD are at higher risk for emotional problems, including anxiety and depression. They often begin to realize that the transition to adulthood or college is looming, and begin to stress about the future. Because they are still very impulsive, 'psych ache' and emotional agitation can lead them to harm themselves. Suicide is often a very impulsive act, and one of the biggest predictors is a person's level of agitation. Kids who are not sleeping, are emotionally distressed, who use substances, and have access to lethal means (especially firearms) are at risk for suicide. A lot of parents assume that emotional problems are just part of being a teenager. If your child's behavior changes significantly at any point, it is essential to seek professional help and remove any easily accessible means of self-harm from your house (especially firearms and prescription drugs)! Taking a 'wait and see' attitude can be deadly.

COLLEGE AND BEYOND

- Write papers
- Read to master material independently
- Manage course/work expectations
- Make strategic plans to complete projects
- Maintain positive relationships with people in authority positions
- Develop close relationships with peers/romantic partners
- Maintain personal health and hygiene (may include obtaining birth control)
- Earn money and budget finances
- Meet deadlines

What may be different with ADHD:

College is often harder for students with ADHD because of their executive functioning difficulties. College is all about executive functioning. Many very smart students are unsuccessful at college because they fail to do basic things like go to class, read the syllabus, or give themselves enough time to do important assignments. The good news is that there is a lot of help to be had. Colleges want your child to succeed. At college, there are supports in place for students who know how to access them. There are resident assistants, professors, friends, advisors and free mental health care for students. Students with a documented disability can get academic support from the college's Disability Support Services office on campus. Fortunate students work with college counselors who know which colleges offer the best disability support programs. If your child will need support, evaluating the support programs of each college is a very important consideration in deciding where to attend.

While college initially seems like high school with more free time, young people have to learn how to be college students. It is essential for students with ADHD that they not miss class. So many students begin missing a class here or there, only to find that their attendance problems lead them to fall behind too fast to catch up. Students with ADHD should take freshman year as easy as possible. They may take a reduced credit load or hold off on harder courses until they are sophomores.

Many students with ADHD want to stop using their accommodations at college. This is a huge mistake for most of them. The support from the Disability Support Services office is critical. College students often fail to recognize how fast little problems build into big ones. For the first year, they need to develop close relationships with counselors, advisors, and disability support staff to keep them on track. It is far easier to prevent problems than it is to get off academic probation, or worse, to drop out in the freshman year.

Many very smart students are unsuccessful at college because they fail to do basic things like go to class, read the syllabus, or give themselves enough time to do important assignments.

ADHD'S IMPACT ON
YOU AND YOUR FAMILY

CHAPTER FOUR:

COPING WITH 'BUTTON-PUSHING' BEHAVIORS

We know that the behaviors of ADHD children are not intentionally malicious, disobedient or annoying. Still, while you can take some behaviors in stride, others make your blood boil. That's why we need to talk about 'Button-Pushing' behaviors.

A 'BUTTON PUSHER' IS A BEHAVIOR THAT EVOKES A STRONG REACTION FOR YOU

Button pushers are behaviors that make us mad or hurt our feelings – or both. They can make us feel powerless, or even sad. These are things your kid does that make you feel like your head is about to explode. Or behaviors that give you that horrible sinking feeling in the pit of your stomach. Or behaviors that have you struggling to hold back tears.

> ### These behaviors 'push our buttons' not because of what the child actually does, but because of who <u>we</u> are.

We all respond irrationally to 'button pushers.'
Our emotions take over and we react – sometimes *overreact*.

> FOR EXAMPLE: imagine a mom comes home from a hard day at work to find the sofa full of greasy snack crumbs. Leaving crumbs on the sofa does not seem like a big deal to her child. He looks at her with a dumfounded expression as she starts 'going nuclear.'
>
> But maybe seeing those crumbs reminds her of how much she'd love to buy some nice furniture like her sister has, but she can't because she has kids. Maybe she remembers the time she heard her mother-in-law whisper her house was "filthy!" Maybe she just spent her entire day off cleaning up the house instead of doing anything fun. Perhaps she just paid $500 to an exterminator to get rid of bugs.

Button pushers are behaviors that make us mad or hurt our feelings – or both. They can make us feel powerless, or even sad. These are things your kid does that make you feel like your head is about to explode.

FAMILY FOCUS

"I've tried everything! I've done sticker charts, time outs, bribes, punishment, ignoring. He can push my buttons and drive me to tears sometimes. On a couple dark days, I even tried spanking. Nothing worked. My husband was dead set against his kid needing therapy, but I was falling apart. I had to put my foot down, and we found a therapist. The first one just wanted to talk about everybody's feelings so we tried another one. I wasn't going to give up on it. I love my son's therapist. He's been a lifesaver. I think sometimes he's saved my marriage as well as my relationship with my son."

The mom's strong reaction comes from feelings almost totally unrelated to the actual behavior itself. If we 'unpack' the feelings in the example, we can see the parent may be feeling:

- Shame
- Anger
- Insulted
- Demoralized

So when the parent subsequently 'goes nuclear,' she is not really reacting to the actual situation, but *to the feelings and associations it evokes.*

DIFFERENT PEOPLE HAVE DIFFERENT BUTTON PUSHERS

If you are married or a co-parent, you might find that the behaviors that make you furious might seem trivial – or even endearing – to your spouse. This can create fertile ground for fights. On a positive note, it can mean it's time for parents to work together to 'tag team' for a bit so the upset parent can recover.

Here is a list of typical button pushers:
- Cursing
- Fighting
- Bullying
- Mistreating siblings
- Mistreating pets
- Ignoring you/your spouse
- Breaking/damaging possessions
- Taking risks (dangerous behavior)
- Back talking or sassiness
- Impolite table manners
- Demanding presents/privileges excessively
- Sloppiness
- Whining
- Throwing tantrums
- Flashing/showing private parts
- Making crude jokes or using toilet humor
- Being selfish/resisting sharing
- Demanding you do things for them that they should be able to do themselves
- Poor hygiene – resisting cleaning teeth, body, fingernails
- Resisting helping out or pitching in/trying to get out of work
- Talking incessantly
- Lying
- Demanding your attention at all times
- Having toileting accidents (well after training is complete)
- Being too wild
- Crying over small things/being 'overly dramatic'
- Dressing in a provocative or slovenly manner

WHAT'S THE KEY TO STOPPING YOURSELF FROM 'GOING NUCLEAR'?

The answer lies in mindfulness. If you are aware of which of your child's behaviors push your buttons, you can make a conscious choice about how to react, instead of losing control.

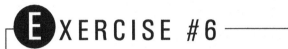

XERCISE #6

LEARNING TO TELL 'RATIONAL BRAIN' FROM 'EMOTIONAL BRAIN' REACTIONS

Before beginning, you and your spouse/co-parent may want to go through the list of button pushers on the opposite page and compare which of these trigger 'nuclear' reactions for each of you.

Now, try answering these questions together. Learning to step back enough to see the difference between 'emotional brain' and 'rational brain' reactions can be extremely helpful in getting control when your child – or anyone – engages in behaviors that push your buttons.

1. **BUTTON PUSHER: Having to work hard to get and keep your child's attention**
   - Is having to work to get your child's attention a button pusher for you?
   - What goes through your mind when it happens?
   - What does it make you feel (ignored, blown-off, out of control)?
   - How likely are you to lose your temper in response?

   What your emotional brain says:
   These kids don't appreciate me! I'm just a servant to them who they can treat like dirt! I'm sick of it and I'm going to show them whose boss!

   Let your rational brain speak instead:
   I'm aware that kids with ADHD need more than the normal level of stimulation, not just to pay attention, but to even feel comfortable. That's why stimulant medications work – they stimulate the areas of the brain that are under-aroused so a child can exert more control. I know that I have to work hard to get and keep my child's attention, but it's not willful behavior. It's simply a symptom of ADHD.

   (continued)

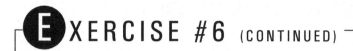

EXERCISE #6 (CONTINUED)

2. **BUTTON PUSHER: Hyperactivity**
   - Is your child's activity level a button pusher for you?
   - What goes through your mind when it happens?
   - What does it make you feel?
   - How likely are you to lose your temper in response?

What your emotional brain says:

This kid is driving me crazy! My father-in-law was right – he's totally spoiled! I'm taking his bike for a month, and I don't care if he cries about it!

Let your rational brain speak instead:

With schools cutting recess and forcing kids into long periods of seatwork, it's frustrating for my child. He needs a lot of opportunities to move so he can feel comfortable, especially on school days. Of course he has extra energy to burn.

3. **BUTTON PUSHER: Impulsive Behavior**
   - Is your child's impulsivity a button pusher for you?
   - What goes through your mind when it happens?
   - What does it make you feel (angry, embarrassed, out of control, jealous)?
   - How likely are you to lose your temper in response?

What your emotional brain says:

This kid is a menace! I can't leave her alone for a second! She acts like a two-year-old! No wonder nobody wants to play with her.

Let your rational brain speak instead:

ADHD makes it hard for her to put on the brakes. She probably did not think through what would happen before she acted. If she did, she probably couldn't stop herself.

EXERCISE #7

CHANGING THE WAY YOU REACT TO BUTTON PUSHERS

Below, we've repeated the list common button pushers. Remember that these are things many children do at their worst moments, not just kids with ADHD. However, given their weaknesses with self-control, kids with ADHD may do these things more often, or well past the age when they are expected.

1. **Circle the behaviors that really push your buttons the most (the ones that really provoke strong feelings):**

    - Cursing
    - Fighting
    - Bullying
    - Mistreating siblings
    - Mistreating pets
    - Ignoring you/your spouse
    - Breaking/damaging possessions
    - Taking risks (dangerous behavior)
    - Back talking or sassiness
    - Impolite table manners
    - Demanding presents/privileges excessively
    - Sloppiness
    - Whining
    - Throwing tantrums
    - Flashing/showing private parts
    - Making crude jokes or using toilet humor
    - Being selfish/resisting sharing
    - Demanding you do things for them that they should be able to do themselves
    - Poor hygiene – resisting cleaning teeth, body, fingernails
    - Resisting helping out or pitching in/trying to get out of work
    - Talking incessantly
    - Lying
    - Demanding your attention at all times
    - Having toileting accidents (well after training is complete)
    - Being too wild
    - Crying over small things
    - Dressing in a provocative or slovenly manner

    (continued)

EXERCISE #7 (CONTINUED)

2. **Pick one.** Imagine a time when your child did this behavior recently – and it provoked strong feelings. Remember that instance from start to finish as best as you can.

   My child really pushed my buttons when:

   WAKING ME UP A 3AM FOR AN

   ENTIRE WEEK AND REFUSING TO

   GO BACK TO THEIR ROOM.

3. **Now replay the memory,** paying close attention to what your *emotional* brain thought:

   • What was going through your mind? _ANGER : WHY S,_
     INSENSITIVE?
   • What did you feel? _FRUSTRATED_
   • How did you handle the situation? _YELLING_
   • Without criticizing yourself, but accepting that nobody is perfect, how do you feel about your response? _NOTHING I CAN DO_
     WHEN IT'S 3AM.

4. **Now replay the memory once more.** This time, practice noticing your *rational* brain response. Imagine yourself like a coach doing a post-mortem on a scrimmage. Try to analyze what happened and why. Your rational brain should be able to identify the ABCs (**Antecedent, Behavior, Consequence**). Your rational brain recognizes why the behavior occurred, or at least can recognize a possible logical explanation.

   Antecedent _POOR SELF CONTROL TO STAY IN BED_

   Behavior _COME IN AT 3AM_

   Consequence _WAKE ENTIRE FAMILY_

EXERCISE #7 (CONTINUED)

5. **Now ask yourself, "If I could go back in time ..."**
   - What would your rational brain have told you to do?
   - Could you have prevented the button-pushing behavior by changing the antecedents?
   - Could you have redirected the child to more tolerable behavior?
   - Would you enact the same consequences if you could do it again?

   Record your thoughts:

   NOTHING I CAN DO.

   _____

6. **What do you think could help you avoid having your 'buttons pushed' next time?**

   NOTHING,

CHAPTER FIVE:

HELPING YOUR CHILD MEET THE CHALLENGES OF ADHD

With ADHD, your child may face challenges in seven key areas:

1. Attention control
2. 'Sleepy brain'
3. Impulse control
4. Emotional regulation
5. Motivation
6. Social relationships
7. Executive functioning

In this chapter, we'll look at each of these areas in terms of what issues typically arise, how your child may respond, and how you can help your child harness her own unique strengths to meet these challenges successfully at home, at school and in the community.

FAMILY FOCUS

"Every week I'd get a phone call from school. On a good week, I get one or two. On a bad week, they'd tell me to come pick him up. The stuff he's doing is not really all that bad or dangerous, I think they just want to get him to go away. Over time, it was like if he sneezed wrong they were throwing a fit about how bad he is. They actually said that they wouldn't let him go to recess unless I came to supervise him. I was committed to Catholic school for my children, so I tried to make it work, but that was the last straw."

CHALLENGE #1: ATTENTION CONTROL _____

Compared to people their same age, those with ADHD have trouble activating, sustaining, and controlling attention.

ADHD is poorly named because it does not mean that the person cannot pay attention. Kids with ADHD can pay attention, often very well, when their brain's attentional system is engaged. The problem is exerting *control* over attention. Some researchers, like Dr. Russel Barkley, consider the primary disorder underlying ADHD symptoms is this inability to control focus, impulses, and ignore distractions.

Not only is it harder to activate the attentional system, it is harder for the child to sustain attention.

EXAMPLES OF BEHAVIORS YOU MIGHT SEE

No action.

For kids with ADHD, their brains do not 'activate' the attentional system as easily as typical peers. You might find yourself saying things like "put your shoes on" 50 times a morning. Your child hears you and understands the meaning of your words, but does not act.

Fatigue or distraction.

Not only is it harder to activate the attentional system, it is harder for the child to sustain attention. The system may be activated (e.g. "everybody start your worksheets now"), but may soon fatigue or become distracted (e.g. "Aidan, it's been 10 minutes and you've only done two problems!").

Excellent attention – sometimes even better than kids without ADHD.

Kids with ADHD need more intense stimulation to activate the attentional system and keep it active. So, when you put a child with ADHD in a highly stimulating situation, you quickly see that his attentional system can work just fine (maybe even better than his peers!). Video games provide that perfect mix of high stimulation with reward. In fact, video games often offer one of the few situations where a child with ADHD actually feels really comfortable. This is why kids with ADHD are at higher risk for addiction or abuse of video games – they are intensely rewarding to their brains.

Hyperfocus.

For many kids with ADHD, the intensity of their attention is actually a big part of the problem. Psychologists call this hyperfocus. Hyperfocus occurs when a child's attention is so intensely engaged it becomes hard for them to shift it. Once activities like video games, LEGOs, drawing, or imaginary play engage the child's attention, it sticks! Daydreams can be a culprit too, and kids are naturally prone to daydream about intense interests such as Star Wars, Pokémon, or Harry Potter. It is so hard to focus on day to day classroom activities when your imagination is so much more engaging!

Kids with ADHD have immature ability to divide their attention (e.g. to pay attention when you call them for dinner). They have more trouble exerting control over it, which psychologist refer to as 'shifting' attention. In this example, the child's attention is so engaged by the video game that they may hear you calling, but not be able to exert enough control to take steps to turn off the game. Kids may also not appear to hear you at all, even if you are in the same room yelling. It is hard for a parent to understand that the child is not actually ignoring you. Most of the time, when the child 'snaps' out of it, they are surprised to find an angry parent or teacher standing over them. Remind yourself that they don't do this on purpose. It makes no more sense to take it personally than it does to blame a car for being slow to start on a cold day.

Trouble modulating their attention.

Kids with ADHD also have immature ability to modulate their level of engagement. Unlike most of us, they can't force themselves to pay attention as well as same-aged peers (like to a boring school lesson). They also can't stop paying attention to something as easily as their peers (like to a fly buzzing around the classroom or a siren wailing off in the distance).

Less aware of fluctuations in attention.

Everyone's attention fluctuates. While you read, for example, your attention wanders around the page or dips into associations you're having about the information. We all know that lapses happen while we drive, but we are rarely conscious of our lapses in attention until something activates our attentional system (like a deer leaping out in front of our car). The difference is that the person with ADHD is less aware of these fluctuations, and even less able to bring attention back to what is most important. This is why many students with ADHD struggle with reading comprehension. They are fine readers of words and sentences, they just can't control their attention well enough to process all the information in the text. It is also why individuals with ADHD are at higher risk for motor vehicle accidents.

Kids may not appear to hear you, even if you are in the same room yelling.

41

HOW OTHERS MIGHT REACT

Noticing that the child can pay attention to some things, less informed people will conclude that the child is lazy or oppositional. Keep in mind, it is not that he's choosing not to pay attention: children with ADHD can no more stop having symptoms and behaviors of ADHD than a person can will away his allergies.

HOW TO HELP YOUR CHILD

1. To help educate people who think a child's lack of attention control is willful, many parents use a statement that goes something like this...

    My child's brain needs higher levels of stimulation in order to
    pay attention and sustain attention than other children do.
    When his brain gets the right level of stimulation, he does fine.

2. What *can* your child pay attention to without a lot of effort
    (list at *least* 3 things):

    TV

    LEGOS

    CARS/ PLANES/ VEHICLES

    Now, think about what those things/activities have in common – these will be the keys to engaging your child's attention! (e.g., "these activities all involve ...." or "these activities take place when my child is ...."

    Did you find common elements? Finish these statements:

    My child can focus on things that are _____

    _____

    My child has the easiest time paying attention when _____

    _____

    In order to engage his attention, my child needs _____

    _____

3. Now, list types of activities that trigger hyperfocus in your child (that intense focus that is hard to shift away from):

    _____

    _____

    _____

What do these activities have in common?

_____

_____

_____

4. Now list at least three things that your child struggles to focus on (think of three things inside of school, then three things outside of school):

_____

_____

_____

What do these things/activities have in common? These are your keys to avoiding triggers and trouble spots:

My child struggles to focus on things that are _____

_____

My child has the hardest time focusing when _____

_____

In order to engage his attention, my child needs to avoid _____

_____

IN CONCLUSION:

Watch for signs of what engages your child's attention. As a parent, you should know what elements have to be there for your kid to be fully engaged. Also notice what sorts of activities trigger problematic hyperfocus. Remember that hyperfocus can be a great asset – people like computer programmers and surgeons excel because of this ability. Be ready to communicate to others exactly what your child needs in the environment to focus and to avoid problematic hyperfocus. Make sure to rehearse a 3-line description so you can make your point to other people clearly and confidently!

We imagine that if a child is hyper, his brain is going a million miles a minute. That is incorrect.

CHALLENGE #2: UNDER-AROUSAL ('SLEEPY BRAIN') _____

Typical activities that keep most children engaged can feel boring or frustrating to kids with ADHD. Why? Their brains are under-aroused. They need more stimulation just to feel ok. Your average classroom sets them up for failure.

If you have a hyper child leaping on the living room sofa, it's hard to think of her as under-aroused – but that under-arousal is what is thought to be causing that sensation-seeking behavior. We imagine that if a child is hyper, his brain is going a million miles a minute. That is incorrect. The under-aroused brain craves stimulation! It takes more stimulation to activate the attentional system than for a regular child. For children with inattentive type ADHD, it can feel like a lot of work trying to activate their attentional system and keep it active (especially when you're trying to get them ready for school on a busy morning).

Today's classroom demands that children sit still for long periods of time and passively absorb information. What a mismatch for our kids with ADHD! Typical children without ADHD can generally suppress their urges to move during the school day. Most kids can sit still well enough to meet the demands of the classroom, but most would say it is not fun to have to do so. The difference for our kids with ADHD is that they cannot suppress these urges as well. So what do they do? They fidget. They rock in their chairs. They wander the room. They drop their pencils. They talk to their neighbor. They blurt out answers or talk too loud. They touch or bump other kids. They chew their shirt collars. In short, they do anything they can to alleviate that need for more stimulation. Their under-aroused or 'sleepy' brains will find ways to get the stimulation they need.

EXAMPLES OF BEHAVIORS YOU MIGHT SEE

- Chewing (pencils, clothing or hair most often)
- Dropping pencils and markers (or utensils at meals)
- Playing with objects
- Getting up and wandering
- Frequent trips to the bathroom or pencil sharpener
- Picking at skin or fingernails
- Calling out/interrupting
- Chatting
- Climbing/jumping (where you're not supposed to)
- Invading others' personal space
- Tapping feet/pencils
- Kicking chair legs
- Swinging book bags or lunch bags while waiting in line
- Talking or touching others in the hallway (when you're supposed to be silent)
- Class Clown behaviors (attention seeking, trying to get others to laugh)
- Singing, talking, or making noises (often the sound effects of his imaginary story playing in his head)
- Checking her phone at inappropriate times
- Sneaking a chance to read or draw

HOW OTHERS MIGHT REACT

Teachers or others may understandably find such behaviors annoying. They may believe the behaviors are intentional and take disciplinary actions. Other people tend to assume the child is doing these things on purpose. They often assume that the child is doing them purposefully to annoy others or to gain attention. Keep in mind that unless teachers understand the 'sleepy brain' aspect of ADHD, they may be affronted at any idea that their classroom is 'under-stimulating.'

HOW TO HELP YOUR CHILD

1. **Help people understand what's going on.**
    Make it clear that ADHD is a brain-functioning disorder and that your child's stimulation-seeking behaviors are not deliberate: they are symptoms of a bored brain. They literally just *happen*. Kids are often unaware that they are doing them!

2. **Try raising awareness of stimulation-seeking behaviors.**
    Imagine having someone yell at you out of the blue for doing something you weren't even aware you were doing. It happens to our kids *every day*. It's not a surprise that so many of our children are anxious or discouraged given how much negative feedback they get. Parents and teachers can help reverse this by gently calling attention to the behaviors *before* they start to cause disruption or negative consequences.

3. **Look for ways to add *positive* stimulation.**
    How many of these behaviors do you think would improve with extra movement built into your child's day? In many cases, the severity of ADHD symptoms could be greatly reduced by changing the environment. Adding in more opportunities to exercise would make a world of difference for all kids, not just ones with ADHD.

Keep in mind that unless teachers understand the 'sleepy brain' aspect of ADHD, they may be affronted at any idea that their classroom is 'under-stimulating.'

Negative consequences are less effective because kids with ADHD don't have full power to 'put on the brakes.'

CHALLENGE #3:
IMPULSE CONTROL AND BEHAVIORAL REGULATION _____

Kids with ADHD are famous for acting without thinking. Why? Because their under-aroused brains can't 'put on the brakes.'

Unlike other animals, humans are capable of metacognition (thinking about thinking, thinking about behavior). We can plan and evaluate our behavior, as well as reflect on it later. Our remarkable brains let us travel through time, from the past to the present, and through what we predict the future will be like. We can do so at will as part of metacognition. Metacognitive abilities mature with age. Children with ADHD have immature metacognition, which often means they are pretty clueless about their own behavior. It is our job to help them make wise choices.

EXAMPLES OF BEHAVIORS YOU MIGHT SEE

Because children with ADHD are often less aware of their own behavior (remember their metacognitive immaturity), they are often surprised by consequences. Their under-aroused brain doesn't stop to consider what is going to happen in the future (what psychologists call 'prospection').

Even if they do pause to consider consequences, they have immature capacity to change course. ***This is why negative consequences are LESS EFFECTIVE*** for kids with ADHD than they are for other kids.

HOW OTHERS MIGHT REACT

Most adults pay attention only to the behavior and the consequence, not what may have triggered it. Parents and teachers, particularly when we are not at our best – when we are Hungry, Angry, Lonely, Tired (HALT), over-focus on the consequences. We tend to have 'knee jerk' reactions to how the child's behavior makes us feel, so we do something we think will make the child stop – anything from redirecting, to criticizing or even yelling. But as we just learned above, negative consequences are less effective because kids with ADHD don't have full power to 'put on the brakes.'

You may find that adults, particularly adults who have not raised children themselves (or have not done so for many years) often have distorted perceptions about what is typical kid behavior. *Adults are quick to decide a child must have acted deliberately.* Grown-ups often ascribe adult levels of sophistication to children's behavior – such as imaging a child is deliberately manipulative. This is true even about teachers or other professionals who should know better.

It is important to communicate to the adults in your child's life that many of his unwanted behaviors are:

- **Not** deliberate
- **Not** planned
- **Not** thought through
- **Not** intended to upset/annoy/anger/provoke other people
- **Not** something he can control

THE *NEW* ABCs OF ADHD

Though a child's behavior may seem random or chaotic, behavior is not all that hard to predict if you know the triggers. Behavior is also not that hard to understand once it has happened – if you know what to look for.

Psychologists are trained to think of the ABCs of behavior. Viewing your child's behavior in these same terms helps improve your understanding of what's going on and the best way to respond. Here are the **ABC**s:

- **A**ntecedent (what triggered that particular behavior at that particular time?)
- **B**ehavior (what did the person do?)
- **C**onsequences (what happened to the child after she did the behavior? Was she rewarded, relieved, punished, ignored?)

We cannot expect that a negative consequence will change behavior for a child with ADHD the way it will for a non-disabled child.

I'm not saying we shouldn't have consequences for unwise or hurtful choices! Children need to learn to respect adult authority. In fact, children are more likely to feel calm in the hands of someone who can enforce limits. Most importantly, they need to learn the skills to make wise choices. Children with ADHD who correct their disruptive behavior are at a great disadvantage. So we can't ignore disruptive behavior, we just have to be smart about how we work to change it.

WHY DID YOU DO THAT?

If you ask children with ADHD, "why did you do that?" you'll find they know the rules. They understand they're not supposed to swing their book bag, run in the hall, or cut their own hair. They know what sorts of behaviors get you in trouble and consequences like getting sent to the principal's office or cut from the team. They can tell you what their teacher likes and does not like. They know that if they drop their tablet computer on the ground one more time you're going to take it away for the whole week (and then go and do it anyway . . .).

But for kids with ADHD, knowing information and making a wise choice are two different things.

Kids with ADHD just can't act on their wise knowledge when an urge strikes (something they have in common with teenagers!). They don't get that burst of 'signal anxiety' that warns them to 'put on the breaks.' 'Signal anxiety' is that little jolt of adrenaline we get when we need to pay attention to something, like a toddler reaching for a hot curling iron. Our brain's alert center detects that something needs paying attention to, and sends signals to the parts of our brain that control our bodies to mobilize a response. In other words, we realize that something needs doing (signal anxiety) and we take steps to do something (something that we believe will relieve that anxiety).

Signal anxiety helps keep us out of trouble. But what if we didn't have it? We would have a hard time avoiding and fixing problems in our lives. We would be more likely to make foolish choices!

Kids with hyperactive type ADHD often misbehave because they simply cannot control their impulses. For children with inattentive type ADHD, forgetfulness or carelessness, not callousness, are often at the root of their behavior issues. Their brain's attentional system does not send out that helpful "Hey! Stop and THINK!" message that helps keep us out of trouble.

So, for kids with ADHD, we need to pay **MORE** attention to the *antecedents* and the *behavior* itself than to the *consequences*. Let's look at the types of consequences:

NATURAL CONSEQUENCES

Here are some of the natural negative consequences for our children's unwanted behaviors ('natural' meaning that an adult does not deliberately do something aversive/unpleasant in order to change the child's behavior):

- Low grades
- Poor academic performance
- Peer rejection
- Negative relationships with teachers
- Losing/ruining valued possessions
- Missing out on something good
- Discomfort
- Getting hurt
- Failure to reach personal goals or to achieve desired outcomes

DELIBERATE CONSEQUENCES

Here are examples of deliberate negative consequences adults often enact with the goal of changing behavior. Deliberate negative consequences are intended to be aversive or unpleasant:

- Time-outs (temporary removal from the activity)
- Shaming/humiliating
- Yelling
- Criticism
- Taking 'points' away/putting the child on a different behavior 'level' (e.g. red on a red/yellow/green system)
- Taking away a possession
- Taking away a privilege (includes taking recess, 'specials' or excluding the child from fun activities)
- Isolating the child to a separate part of the classroom/lunchroom
- Giving extra work/chores/unpleasant tasks
- Causing physical pain

PUNISHMENT VS. DISCIPLINE

It has been my observation that the happiest kids are the ones whose parents set limits and enforce rules. Focusing on consequences, however, does not work as well for any child, and especially for kids with ADHD.

Sometimes, consequences can even take the form of punishment. Punishment is taking deliberate action to cause discomfort in the form of an aversive (unwanted) experience. If you look at the list of Deliberate Consequences, many of these are punishments. Extensive research shows that punishment is not only less effective than other ways of disciplining, but also tends to increase aggression in children. Plus, as old punishments lose effect, it leads to harsher and harsher punishments. No parent wants to go down that road.

Am I saying a child should never be punished? That's not realistic. Some situations warrant an unpleasant consequence. The problem is that as parents we over-rely on punishments. I'm saying that when we look at our 'toolkit' for teaching our children how to behave, punishment is one of our least effective tools. If our goal is to help a child learn to be a wise person with strong morals, we have to teach self-discipline.

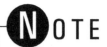

NOTE

Not all unwanted behaviors are about seeking stimulation. Some behaviors are inconsiderate, self-destructive or hurtful to others.

Not all children with ADHD engage in such behaviors. Plenty of kids without ADHD are very capable of being mean or disruptive too.

There is a difference when a child hurts his friend accidentally because he tackled him too roughly during play and when a child intentionally body slams another out of anger. Aggressive and manipulative behaviors tend to come from emotional discomfort. Children who feel safe, valued, cared for, and understood, do not generally engage in hurtful behaviors on purpose.

THE SECRET IS TO TEACH CHILDREN SOMETHING NEW

Discipline comes from an old word that meant *teaching*, not punishing. Where to start? We can teach children not to do a specific behavior (e.g. "Stop kicking the chair legs!"). That is not so hard. But the child will still have the same need that generated the behavior in the first place – the same boredom, desire for attention, frustration, sadness, or intense desire to move. Remember, every behavior occurs for a reason. It serves some purpose for the person doing it – it is an attempt to satisfy a need! This is why teachers and parents often notice that unwanted behaviors don't go away, they just morph into other ones. For example, kicking the chair legs may stop, but then the child may start getting up out of his seat or tapping his pencil.

Look back at the list of deliberate consequences. Do any of those consequences teach the child how do to something NEW to replace an unwanted behavior? Some might give the child a chance to calm down, but few on that list teach new skills. *And new skills are what kids with ADHD desperately need.*

HOW TO HELP YOUR CHILD

1. **Learn how to uncover the 'antecedents.'**
    To do this, let's go back to your list of the easy/hard activities and hyperfocus triggers you created earlier (pages 42-43).

    Pick a trigger or activity from your list – something that is difficult for your child to focus on or that is hard for him to shift his attention away from. Ideally, try to pick one that has caused recent problems for your child.

    My child's 'difficult' activity is ___STAYING IN BED___

    This is your 'antecedent.' Now, look at that antecedent and **define what makes this activity hard** or why it triggers your child's behaviors (e.g., is it boring, does it involve sitting still, is it embarrassing, does it make your child anxious?). Write your response below:

    _____

    _____

    Now identify at least one **negative feeling your child experiences** while engaged in this activity (for example, if you picked math worksheets, you might say your child feels frustrated). Write your response below:

    ___Scared?___

    How long can your child tolerate this feeling before she engages in unwanted behaviors?

    ___NOT AT ALL___

> The child will still have the same need that generated the behavior in the first place – the same boredom, desire for attention, frustration, sadness, or intense desire to move.

2. Next, look at the behavior itself.

Put on your 'detective' hat and begin to identify why your child's unwanted behaviors occur or persist. Working through these two lists will help you practice being a 'behavior detective.' This, in turn, will help you sharpen your skills at anticipating or uncovering how specific antecedents trigger(ed) specific behavior.

Start by circling any of the **behaviors** below that finish the sentence, *'In order to get more stimulation in an under-stimulating situation, my child is likely to engage in:*

- Chewing (pencils, clothing or hair most often)
- Dropping pencils and markers (or utensils at meals)
- Playing with objects
- Getting up and wandering
- Frequent trips to the bathroom or pencil sharpener
- Picking at skin or fingernails
- Calling out/interrupting
- Chatting
- Climbing/jumping (where you're not supposed to)
- Invading others' personal space
- Tapping feet/pencils
- Kicking chair legs
- Swinging book bags or lunch bags while waiting in line
- Talking or touching others in the hallway (when you're supposed to be silent)
- Class Clown behaviors (attention seeking or trying to get others to laugh)
- Singing, talking, or making noises (often the sound effects of his imaginary story playing in his head)
- Checking her phone at inappropriate times
- Sneaking a chance to read or draw

Now, look at the next list below. Circle the **emotional response** that completes the sentence, *"In response to emotional discomfort, a child may engage in:"*

- Avoidance (trying to get out of having to do the task)
- Withdrawal (shutting down, daydreaming, fantasizing)
- Escape attempts (finding a way to leave the situation, such as going to the nurse or bathroom)
- Crying/having a tantrum
- Expressing frustration
- Aggression

... begin to identify why your child's unwanted behaviors occur or persist.

3. **Take some of the guesswork out of why behaviors happen and what to expect.**
    Using the work you just did, pick one of the behaviors and fill in the blanks below:

    [Write in the BEHAVIOR] _____

    is most likely to occur after my child has been struggling with [write

    in the ANTECEDENT] _____ .

    After _____ minutes, I believe that my child will try to get relief from

    these uncomfortable feelings, by exhibiting: [WRITE IN EMOTIONAL

    RESPONSE] _____ .

    Help your child become aware of consequences. Think about the particular antecedent and behavior you chose to think about for this section. Try to identify the natural negative consequences and the deliberate negative consequences your child experiences when he does the behavior.

    When my child does _____

    He is trying to get _____

    He experiences natural negative consequences like _____

    _____

    And adults inflict negative consequences like _____

    _____

4. **Get ahead of behaviors.**
    Consequences for children with ADHD must address their specific weaknesses – they need to learn self-control. The best consequences teach what psychologist Dr. Alan Kazdin calls 'Positive Opposite' behaviors. A positive opposite behavior *teaches a child a new behavior for satisfying a need*. The trick is that the 'positive opposite' behavior has to be incompatible with the undesirable behavior – for example, a child can't kick his chair legs and hold his legs out straight at the same time.

    Go back to the list of antecedents you created. Match them up with behaviors and then think of a possible 'Positive Opposite' behavior. Remember that the 'positive opposite' behavior has to satisfy the same need that the original behavior did. SO if the child was engaging in the behavior in order to get more stimulation, you'll need to figure out an acceptable way for the child to get that stimulation.

Here are a few examples and (below) a list of positive opposite activities
to get you started.

ANTECEDENT	BEHAVIOR	POSITIVE OPPOSITE BEHAVIOR
Boring math class	Kicking the chair	Child is given a 'fidget'
Standing in line a long time	Swinging the lunch bag	Child is asked to do jumping jacks instead

Below is a list of changes to the antecedent environment and positive opposite activities that work well to satisfy the need for more stimulation. These are changes you can make at home and school to provide kids with ADHD more stimulation (and better focus!). You can ask for these in your child's IEP/504 Plan or Learning Support Plan in an independent school.

'Positive Opposites' for increasing the level of stimulation.

- Using a fidget (small object to hold and manipulate)
- Chewing gum (better for older kids) or 'chewy tubes' (best for kids under 5)
- Movement breaks
- Exercise breaks
- Getting a drink of water
- Sitting on a yoga ball or sensory chair cushion
- Giving kids light-up or vibrating timers to prompt attention
- Do rote skill practice using fun computer software
- Have kids type written responses
- Allow children to stand at their desks or lie on the floor to work
- Work outside
- Event based/problem-solving based learning
- Cooperative learning (working in a group)

CHALLENGE #4: EMOTIONAL REGULATION _____

Kids with ADHD have trouble controlling their emotions and find it very hard to ignore emotional discomfort.

Our brains only have so much 'bandwidth' available for processing information. Our emotions help us determine where it is most important to pay attention (do we pay attention to our email or the crying baby?). In children with ADHD, the part of the brain that calms down strong emotions (the prefrontal cortex) is less active. This results in an immature ability to control emotions.

EXAMPLES OF BEHAVIORS YOU MIGHT SEE

Higher highs, lower lows.

Kids with hyperactivity tend to have 'higher highs' where they can become wild (e.g. tackling friends when they win a soccer game). They can also have 'lower lows' where they fall apart over seemingly trivial events (e.g. throwing a tantrum when they lose a soccer game).

Low resilience.

Children with ADHD find it hard to ignore emotional discomfort. Things that most children 'bounce back' from easily can really discourage them. This is one reason they are more vulnerable to anxiety and depression than most children.

Difficulty persevering.

Children with ADHD who feel emotionally overwhelmed can find it hard to 'go with the flow.' Small 'triggers' can hijack them. Their frustration can hit like a tidal wave. Kids with ADHD have a harder time persisting through frustration and sticking with strenuous mental work. This is part of why they have such a hard time persevering through challenges. Their trouble persevering in the face of frustration often gets labeled as laziness or lack of motivation. Recent research on the quality of 'grit' or persisting through obstacles, indicates that grit is a better predictor of success than intelligence in some situations. Children with ADHD are thus at higher risk for under-achieving because they cannot tolerate frustration as well.

Under-reaction.

Children with ADHD can, conversely, be under-reactive. Situations that SHOULD cause stress do not phase them. Remember the bit about 'signal anxiety'? Our brains normally do a great job alerting us to pay attention to something important and then mobilizing a response. Some level of stress is essential, or else we would never get out of bed or pay the mortgage. Kids with ADHD do not get the 'signal' to get worried.

For example, the teen who is flunking out of school, but does not see why she can't spend each night staying out with her friends. Remember, the under-aroused, 'sleepy brain' needs a stronger trigger to alert the attentional system.

NOTE

As researcher Dr. Russel Barkley famously noted, *children with ADHD tend to be about three years less emotionally mature than same aged peers.*

So-called 'signal anxiety' – that helpful jolt of adrenaline that spurs us to take action – never happens for them. That teenager has some awareness that she's failing, and knows intellectually that failing could mean summer school, but right now? She's focused on how much she wants to go to the mall and cannot see why you will not let her go. Some people with ADHD seem to drift through life unperturbed by their troubles. Of course that's fine until other people get tired of cleaning up after them! This atypical passivity can be a huge source of stress in the family. Parents often differ in how much they want to 'rescue' the child vs. how much to let her learn from experience.

Negative self-concepts.

Children with ADHD receive considerably more negative feedback about themselves than their peers. Imagine how many times during the course of your child's day he receives positive reactions and/or praise. Now consider how many times each day the child receives redirection, criticism, negative feedback or punishment. Researchers who study relationships have found that we need at least five positive encounters for every negative one in order to feel good in a relationship. Most children, particularly those with hyperactive type ADHD, fall far short of the positivity they need. It is no surprise they start disliking school earlier. When you learn that you are not one of those 'gold star' kids who can please the teacher, you may soon stop trying.

Anxiety.

ADHD and anxiety disorders often co-occur because both have to do with attention control.

ADHD and anxiety disorders often co-occur because both have to do with attention control. Everyone responds to stress and danger but people vary in how reactive their brains are. Some of us are calm in a crisis, while others panic when we lose our keys. Most of us will calm down pretty quickly after danger has passed, but people with anxiety disorders don't. Their brain keeps paying attention to ideas of danger and worries. Their brains may even blow small worries way out of proportion, sometimes into actual panic attacks. Mental health professionals call these upsetting thoughts 'automatic negative thoughts' – or ANTs. People who can't ignore ANTs are chronically distracted by a stress response that won't go away – even though the stress response is way out of proportion compared to the actual danger.

Impaired memory and concentration.

If a child finds it very hard to control attention, her mind can become so filled with distressing thoughts, worries, fears and other ANTs, that there is not much bandwidth left for getting work done. Anxiety takes energy away from thinking, memory, learning, and concentrating. Add ADHD to the mix, and those distressing thoughts get even harder to ignore. Not only do students with ADHD find it hard to ignore ANTs, they have all the problems of being a kid with ADHD to 'feed' the worries. The good news is that anxiety disorders respond very well to cognitive behavioral therapy and medication. Kids with ADHD can learn to manage their focus and get those ANTs exterminated.

HOW TO HELP YOUR CHILD

1. **Help others (teachers, coaches, other parents) understand** the emotional issues a child with ADHD faces. This can go a long way toward addressing situations before they become too frustrating for your child or they provoke anxiety.

2. **Don't spare the constructive praise.** This doesn't mean giving our children constant praise – far from it. Children can spot phony praise. I'm talking about constructive praise. Research on praise shows us that empty praise ascribes value to the person (You're so smart! You're so talented!) Actually erodes motivation. Constructive praise is directed towards a person's choices. Constructive praise targets actions and choices (You worked very hard today! You didn't give up, even when it got tough!).

3. **Use 'positive regard' to eliminate negative labels.** The best adults in his life will look for what is great about him. They will be realistic about his abilities, expecting him to rise to his best efforts. Too many of our children with ADHD are labeled (remember the difference between labels and diagnoses?). Adults who don't' know any better label them, and afterward, see all of the child's behavior through that distorted lens. It is our job to help kids break out of destructive labels. To read more about this, the book *How to Talk So Kids Will Listen & Listen So Kids Will Talk* gives an excellent 'how to' guide to helping kids break out of roles.

4. **Remember your child may be 'younger on the inside.'** Your child may look a certain age on the outside, but have the emotional maturity of a much younger child. Unfortunately, adults often confuse physical maturity with emotional maturity.

   Your eight-year-old with ADHD may still fall apart crying over a lost soccer game, while his teammates are happily reaching for the orange slices. Your eleven-year-old girl with ADHD may prefer to play with the boys or younger children, because she can't understand the complexities of the 'tween social milieu. Your kids may have tantrums well past the point when most children do. Your teen with ADHD may be shaving, but he still needs organizational help. The important thing is to remember that at any age, children with ADHD may need the same level of support as a much younger child.

It is our job to help kids break out of destructive labels.

CHALLENGE #5: MOTIVATION _____

Because children with ADHD have lower brain levels of the neurotransmitters associated with pleasure, they need bigger, more exciting rewards.

Children with ADHD have a lower response to rewards than other children do. This is due to lower levels of dopamine and norepinephrine in the areas of the brain that get stimulated when we expect or receive pleasure. This means that rewards don't feel as good or exciting. They need bigger, more exciting rewards, which is why traditional motivators like sticker charts don't tend to work very long for kids with ADHD.

EXAMPLES OF BEHAVIORS YOU MIGHT SEE

A focus on instant gratification.

Under-aroused ADHD brains don't get excited about the idea of earning a reward in the future, so they tend to choose instant gratification. Unfortunately, most long-term goals can be achieved only through persistence and hard work — that quality called 'grittiness.' Their weaker 'reward reaction' means they too frequently give up when the going gets tough.

Procrastination.

Students with ADHD find it harder to resist the temptation of choosing satisfaction (the test is not 'til tomorrow, I have plenty of time to play Minecraft). Combined with a weak ability to estimate the time needed to complete a task, they are very vulnerable to procrastination. This often becomes a huge problem (particularly in high school). Students with ADHD often underestimate how much hard work a task will require — that weak awareness of time is a symptom. Their under-aroused brain does not sound the alarm about possible problems on the horizon.

Difficulty with self-motivation.

Most of us self-motivate in one of two ways: We get ourselves excited about the possible reward (I'll ace the test and get into Harvard!). Or, we focus on how much we want to avoid loss and pain (if I fail this test I'll never get into college!). For this to work, giving ourselves these messages needs to set off reactions in the brain and body that trigger behavior changes. Some sort of discrepancy between what we want and what we are experiencing needs to galvanize us to take purposeful action. Kids with ADHD are famous for having goals but not following through to make them happen.

Vulnerability to addictions.
The difference in ADHD brain function (diminished response to rewards coupled with diminished fear of danger) is thought to be a primary reason that people with ADHD are at higher risk for addiction to drugs, alcohol and cigarettes.

HOW OTHERS MIGHT REACT

Young people with ADHD are often criticized for being lazy. It is easy to confuse a lack of persistence with being unmotivated. Many young people with ADHD want to achieve goals, but simply do not know how to do so. Students often get overwhelmed by the daily grind of forcing themselves through their work (remember that sustained mental effort is harder for kids with ADHD, and less rewarding). Children with ADHD have trouble getting excited about the idea of rewards in the future because of neurotransmitter levels – not character flaws.

HOW TO HELP YOUR CHILD

Since students with ADHD struggle to use motivation techniques independently, many need adult help.

- For younger students, Behavior Intervention Plans (called BIPs in schools) help provide rewards to make wise choices more exciting.

- Specialists like tutors and ADHD coaches are often called upon to help high school students through the long slog of assignments.

- Psychotherapy with parent coaching often involves learning better communication skills, routines, and behavior intervention plans.

- Psychotherapy for your child can include individual and/or group treatments to help kids learn how to set and achieve goals.

- Model what you want to see! Show your kids that hard work and perseverance are the path to success by setting a good example.

Many young people with ADHD want to achieve goals, but simply do not know how to do so.

CHALLENGE #6: FORMING GOOD SOCIAL RELATIONSHIPS ___

Children with ADHD may need to learn social skills that many of us develop naturally.

Targeting social skills can have a BIG payoff – perhaps protecting your child from loneliness, anxiety, and depression later on in life.

Many children with ADHD have satisfying social lives. What adults perceive as off-putting 'wildness,' other children may find exciting. There is no reason a child with ADHD cannot be popular and well liked – and many are! Consider the young 'class clowns' who grew up to be entertainers, for example.

For others, ADHD symptoms interfere. The same impulsive behaviors and emotional immaturity that affect their relationships with parents and teachers have negative consequences for their friendships.

You might imagine that social skills are far down on your 'to do' list. I'll suggest that they matter just as much, if not more, than academics. A child who feels accepted has better self-esteem than a child who feels rejected or isolated. Research shows that social rejection or bullying significantly affects our adult mental health. Targeting social skills can have a BIG payoff – perhaps protecting your child from loneliness, anxiety, and depression later on in life (and perhaps getting you a nice future son or daughter in law).

EXAMPLES OF BEHAVIORS YOU MIGHT SEE

- Your child may prefer activities that appeal to younger children, and may not fit in well with same-aged peers.

- Your child may not notice when his behavior is off-putting, annoying, or upsetting.

- Your child may fail to notice social cues/social signals from others.

- Your child may be caught up in her imagination and ignore her peers.

- Your child may play too rough, and may sometimes accidentally hurt others.

- Your child may lose control – crying or having a tantrum in the face of obstacles.

- Your child may say inappropriate or unexpected things.

- Your child may try to engage with other children by being rude or intrusive.

HOW OTHERS MIGHT REACT

Other people may interpret the child's impulsive behavior as deliberate aggression. Your child's impulsivity may be interpreted as deliberately rude or mean. Others may assume your child has not been taught good manners (ouch!). Your child may not be selected by others for friendships or group activities.

HOW TO HELP YOUR CHILD

1. **Social skills may need to be taught.** Children with ADHD may need to learn social skills that many of us develop naturally. Social skills group leaders, speech language pathologists, and psychotherapists can teach these skills.

2. **Be alert to bullying** and address it immediately with teachers and parents.

3. **Help others understand the challenges of ADHD** so that they no longer see behaviors as willfully rude or aggressive.

Your child's impulsivity may be interpreted as deliberately rude or mean. Others may assume your child has not been taught good manners (ouch!).

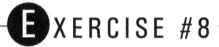 **XERCISE #8**

IS YOUR CHILD LIKE YOU?

For all of us who felt left out or mistreated, we know the pain of social rejection. It can hurt deeply to watch your child go through it.

Remember that list of button pushers (page 32)? Note how many relate to social behavior! Sometimes our children's social problems are the biggest button pushers for us — especially if their social interaction evokes awful memories of our own childhood struggles. Our fear that our child will experience the same social pain we did turns *their* social transgressions into *our* button pushers. This exercise is a good way to look at this.

1. Think back to your own childhood relationships: what were they like?

2. In general, did you have good relationships with teachers and other authority figures?

3. Did you feel accepted and liked by other children?

4. In general, were you able to make and keep friends?

5. Were you a social butterfly? Outsider? Outcast? Popular?

6. Were you an introvert or an extrovert?

7. Is your child like you?

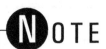

NOTE

Research estimates that about fifty percent of children with ADHD also have specific learning disabilities (neurological differences that impact their achievement in a given area such as language arts or mathematics).

CHALLENGE #7: EXECUTIVE FUNCTIONS _____

Kids with ADHD – even those with high IQs – tend to work harder, not smarter.

Because of their brain's neurological differences, many kids with ADHD will have difficulties in the area of executive functioning. A child's ability to handle Executive Functions has a direct impact on learning and achievement.

Executive functions are brain abilities that allow us to work strategically and efficiently.

You may have heard that these functions are 'housed' in the brain's frontal lobe. Actually, they result from many neural circuits working together across several areas of the brain. The brain's prefrontal cortex receives information from areas that govern emotion, movement, and alertness. It also communicates back to those areas to mediate responses.

Executive functioning in a typical brain: If you think you see a hornet crawling on your shirt, your brain immediately notifies your body to 'fight or flee.' Your Behavioral Inhibition System may kick in, causing you to freeze as you feel adrenaline coursing through your body. The attentional system is now active.

However, you realize that what you thought was a hornet is really just a cricket. Your prefrontal cortex tells the lower regions of your brain to calm down, it was a false alarm. In a well-functioning brain, the body and mind relax.

Executive functioning in an ADHD brain: In an overly anxious ADHD brain, despite the fact that there was no actual threat, the fear of being stung may linger or even intensify. The child may start avoiding outside activities to avoid being scared again.

TWO TYPES OF EXECUTIVE FUNCTIONS: BEHAVIORAL REGULATION AND METACOGNITIVE

Behavioral Regulation: The 'hot' executive functions

The first category is Behavioral Regulation. These are the 'hot' executive functions that allow us to regulate our emotions and behavior, including the ability to:

- **SHIFT:** Focusing our attention on what is most important

- **INHIBIT:** Controlling impulses, ignoring distractions, thinking before acting

- **EMOTIONAL CONTROL:** Calming ourselves down, not getting carried away by strong feelings

If you have the type of child who has hyperactive-impulsive type ADHD, you know how much trouble difficulties with 'hot' executive functions can cause. We see problems with 'hot' executive functions when our kids struggle to follow rules, including the unwritten rules of social interactions. Problems in these areas can also cause our kids to become 'flooded' by strong emotions (frustration, anxiety, anger etc.).

Metacognitive: The 'cool' executive functions

Remember the term metacognition? If not, metacognition is the ability to think about thinking. It refers to our uniquely human ability to approach tasks strategically, plan ahead, and evaluate how well we did. These are the 'cool' executive functions that make school success possible. Problems with these type of executive functions are more likely to become problems in third grade, when tasks get longer and more detailed. Some kids may not have problems with the 'cool' executive functions until they leave the structure of elementary school for the fast pace of middle school.

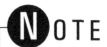

NOTE

Children with Superior IQs and ADHD (often called 'Twice Exceptional' or '2e' kids for short), may actually never have low achievement or significant trouble learning. This does not mean that they don't have ADHD, but that their intelligence is a protective factor.

WHAT DOES EXECUTIVE FUNCTIONING INCLUDE?

Executive functioning covers a broad range of abilities. While researchers differ over how to categorize and define the executive functions, the BRIEF is a behavior rating scale offering a list of functions that seems to generally represent current thinking. The BRIEF (Behavior Regulation Inventory of Executive Functions) was developed by Dr. Gerry Gioia and his colleagues at Children's National Medical Center.

Below is the BRIEF framework of functions. As you read through it, you may immediately see areas of strength and struggle for your child.

- **Initiate:** Starting a task without becoming distracted or overwhelmed

- **Working Memory:** Recalling and recognizing what you have just heard and seen, holding onto that information so you can use it to solve problems

- **Plan/Organize:** Breaking down a task so you can finish it efficiently, working strategically

- **Organize Materials:** Keeping supplies and possessions where you can find them when you need them, coming prepared with the right supplies for the occasion

- **Monitor:** Paying attention to the quality of your own work, detecting errors, making changes when something is not working

In addition to categories included within the BRIEF list, there are two others that are considered important:

- **Time Awareness:** Estimating how much time has passed, predicting how much time something will take, working at the right pace to finish on time

- **Cognitive Efficiency:** Working quickly enough to finish without becoming distracted, keeping the right pace so you can finish without making too many mistakes, knowing when to look at the 'big picture' vs. details

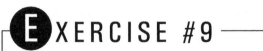

EXERCISE #9

LOOKING AT YOUR OWN CHILD'S EXECUTIVE FUNCTIONING

1. **Behavior Regulation.** Describe a problem your child has in each of these 'hot' areas:

   I see problems with *Shift* when: _____

   _____

   I see problems with *Inhibit* when: _____

   _____

   I see problems with *Emotional Control* when: _____

   _____

2. **Metacognitive.** Take a moment to think about when the 'cool' executive functions are challenging for your child. Homework time is a typical one, especially after second grade. For some children, these difficulties are really only evident in the classroom, but fill in what you know (or ask the teacher!).

   I see difficulties with *Initiate* when:_____

   _____

   I see difficulties with *Working Memory* when: _____

   _____

   I see difficulties with *Plan/Organize* when: _____

   _____

   I see difficulties with *Organize Materials* when:_____

   _____

   I see difficulties with *Monitor* when:_____

   _____

   I see difficulties with *Time Awareness* when: _____

   _____

   I see difficulties with *Cognitive Efficiency* when: _____

   _____

STUDENTS WITH IMMATURE EXECUTIVE FUNCTIONING: THE 'STRATEGY DEFICIENT' LEARNERS

Students with ADHD are often thought of as 'strategy deficient.' They may be bright or even highly gifted, but don't naturally develop strategies for getting things done efficiently. They tend to work harder instead of 'working smarter.'

Our current understanding of the brain tells us that 'strategy-based instruction' is more effective, with teachers going beyond content to teach students how to learn and work strategically.

Strategy-based instruction.
Did you know when teachers teach, they literally rewire a child's brain? Great teaching is, quite literally, transformative. In the old days, teachers taught content. Our current understanding of the brain tells us that 'strategy-based instruction' is more effective, with teachers going beyond content to teach students *how to learn and work strategically.*

Challenges for the ADHD brain.
For most kids, as the frontal lobe matures, higher order thinking tasks seem to unfold naturally, taking them beyond rote procedures to true understanding and allowing them to work smarter, not harder. This doesn't happen in the brains of our kids with learning differences. Their brains have to use considerable resources from the frontal lobe to solve problems that have become fairly automatic for most of their peers. So grade level tasks can feel just plain harder. These kids, even those with high IQs, tend to work *harder, not smarter.* Give them a complex task, and it feels like watching someone tread water instead of swim. They dive right in and exhaust themselves, never getting across the pool to the finish line.

ADHD students have to be taught how to use their brain's executive functioning abilities.

The good news is that decades of research shows the benefits of systematically teaching children to be strategic. This means applying a metacognitive approach. Let's see how this works.

SYSTEM I + SYSTEM II = LEARNING TO BE STRATEGIC

SYSTEM I: Automatic

This is the system in our brain that relies on habit, automatic responses, and minimal contemplation (e.g. reciting the Pledge of Allegiance, driving to work). It is an approach psychologist Dr. Daniel Khaneman referred to as our brain's 'System I.'

System I gives us access to information we can use without giving it much thought at all.

Automatic skills like the multiplication tables and spelling make it possible for students to turn their attention to complex tasks like solving equations or writing an essay. You have a very hard time doing either of those things if you have to stop to think about every component step, so getting rote skills and procedures to the 'System One' level of ease is important.

SYSTEM II: Problem-solving

System II is the system in the brain that snaps into action when there is a novel problem to solve and we need to use *conscious, active* attention (e.g. writing an essay or swerving to avoid a deer in front of the car). Through metacognition, we can *actively decide to engage System II.*

The problem is that most students with ADHD rely on the wrong system at the wrong time.

Children with ADHD are often using System II (the problem-solving system), when they should be able to fall back on System I (the automatic system).

> *For example, a child with ADHD who has never memorized basic addition facts continues to count on his fingers to get the answer.*

This is using System II for what should be an automatic, System I task. Why is that a problem? Using System II takes more energy and focus – something in short supply for our kids with ADHD. Using the wrong system takes more work!

Basic academic skills, the ones that get learned before third grade must all be mastered by third grade in order to 'free up' System II for the heavy-duty content based instruction.

PROBLEMS THAT ARISE WHEN KIDS CHOOSE THE WRONG SYSTEM

Overusing System I:

Students tend to rely on System I as they get older. Why? Because System I is faster and easier. It takes less effort because the information is right there for the brain to access. The result is that students who over-rely on System I are not strategic (remember we called our kids with ADHD 'strategy deficient?').

Instead of sounding the alert that a problem requires a strategy, the under-aroused brain falls back on doing things the same old way. This is why our children's work often looks like little effort was put in, even if they worked very hard.

Using System I to solve a complex problem leads to problems like:

- Misunderstood directions
- Poor task completion
- Careless errors
- Reading text without actually comprehending ('surface' reading)

Overusing System II:

System II is a 'bandwidth hog' that sucks up all the cognitive energy. Imagine trying to solve a quadratic equation if you had to stop and count each step on your fingers! We would all find ourselves hating algebra. Basic academic skills, the ones that get learned before third grade (reading high-frequency words, basic math facts, spelling common words, penmanship) must all be mastered by third grade in order to 'free up' System II for the heavy-duty content-based instruction (science, history, literature, word problems).

SELF-MONITORING

Choosing the wrong System has to do with the brain's ability to pay attention to its own process (metacognition). We call this 'self-monitoring.'

Just as children with ADHD struggle to pay attention to the right things in the world around them, they often fail to give close attention to their own thoughts. Without paying attention to their thoughts, they dive right in – but without a strategy. Their goal too often is to get an unpleasant task done as soon as possible! The result? Underperformance.

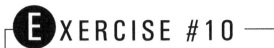

EXERCISE #10

WHEN DOES YOUR CHILD CHOOSE THE WRONG SYSTEM?

1. **Where is your child relying too heavily on System I?** Identify tasks where he seems to be 'phoning it in' or failing to give close attention. Examples might include: writing a paragraph/essay, reading books, multistep math operations or organizing work supplies.

    _____

    _____

    _____

2. **Where is your child relying too heavily on System II?** List examples of situations in which you see your child using lots of mental energy for things that should be automatic, low-effort tasks. Examples might include: cleaning up a messy room, reading words, spelling, or handwriting.

    _____

    _____

    _____

A TALE OF TWO ASSIGNMENTS _____

In the following example, look for:
- Hot Executive functions (emotional self-regulation)
- Cold executive functions (metacognition)
- Using System I for a System II task

Harry has to write an essay. Harry is a middle school biology student with combined type ADHD. This diagnosis means that he is hyperactive, impulsive, and struggles with distractibility. He also has trouble sustaining mental effort as well as persisting through challenges. Though he is as tall as his mother, he is more like an elementary school kid emotionally. Tonight, Harry must write an extended constructed response (roughly a three paragraph answer) explaining why a car is not a living thing. Since his school tries to incorporate writing across curricular areas, this assignment will count both for biology and for English.

SCENARIO ONE: **NO STRATEGY**

DEFICIT: Organization. As luck would have it, Harry left the worksheet with the directions at school (note the deficit in the Executive Function called 'Organization'). Bad luck again, it's only September and Harry does not have the phone number of any friends in his biology class. Third strike: the teacher has not posted the directions on the class webpage. This is going to be quite an evening ...

DEFICIT: Initiation. Harry has great ideas, and can expound on all sorts of topics of great interest to him. Unfortunately, this essay is not about Great White Sharks or soccer, so Harry has spent the past half-hour doing anything and everything except writing (note the deficit in the Executive Function called 'Task Initiation'). So far, he's gotten two snacks, let the dog out and in, put on music, and wandered around the house. He stares at the empty paper until dad finally comes over to help.

DEFICIT: Self-Regulation. Seeing dad's frustrated look, Harry is suddenly in tears.

DEFICIT: Planning and Working Memory. Harry swears he has no idea what to write because he's forgotten the instructions his teacher gave in class that afternoon. Dad grimaces and sits down. They brainstorm some ideas. Dad goes back to his email, hoping Harry is unstuck.

DEFICIT: Task Completion and Self-Monitoring. Eventually, Harry writes three sentences that are about cars and aliens, but does not explain why a car is not alive. Satisfied, he shouts "Done!" and runs off for his post-homework Minecraft time.

Mom and dad start arguing about what to do – should they pull him off the computer and make him redo it? Should they tell him what to write? Punish him? Ground him? Take away the computer? Both know tomorrow night will be more of the same.

SCENARIO TWO: **WITH SYSTEM II**

Now we revisit our friend Harry, but give the story a happy ending.

Imagine that Harry has had a comprehensive psychological evaluation that was shared with his fabulous special education teacher, Ms. Meta. Ms. Meta knows Harry's pattern of strengths and weaknesses. She knows the 6th grade biology class has this assignment due tomorrow, so Harry is already on her 'radar.'

STRATEGY: Organization. She pulls Harry for regular Strategies-Based Instruction in the resource room. First, she has Harry 'activate prior knowledge' by using an online graphic organizer for brainstorming.

STRATEGY: Initiation. Next, she and Harry select their writing strategy, the TREE strategy, which stands for Topic sentence, Reasons, Ending, Examine (*Powerful Writing Strategies for All Students* by Harris and Graham).

STRATEGY: Planning and Working Memory. Harry uses the TREE strategy and the Hamburger Paragraph writing strategy to create a rough draft on his tablet.

STRATEGY: Task Completion and Self-Regulation. Ms. Meta sets a vibrating timer that goes off every two minutes, cuing Harry to monitor his attention. After 15 minutes, she challenges Harry to see how many errors he can find and fix in 120 seconds. Finally, they take one more look at the assignment rubric, making sure his work has met each of the teacher's expectations. The finished work gets emailed to the regular education teacher, not stuffed in the cluttered abyss of Harry's backpack.

When Harry goes home that night, his homework is memorizing a set of vocabulary words. This is a well-defined task that he can do with flashcards and monitoring from dad. After a half hour, it is Minecraft time.

Notice how the strategies-based instruction addressed all of Harry's major Executive Function weaknesses? It was certainly less painful for all involved, and gave Harry a systematic plan for completing the task. Harry's no longer treading water, he's making it to the finish line.

Over time, Harry will internalize these metacognitive strategies so that he needs less and less direct support. That transition to independence is what great interventions are all about! (More on that in our Action Plan).

CHAPTER SIX:

WORKING WITH YOUR CHILD'S STRENGTHS AND WEAKNESSES

Every person is unique, so every person has strengths and weaknesses. Most of your 'average' kids are good at some things and have to work harder at others. Most average kids do not have big 'peaks and valleys.' Instead, they are sort of low-to-high *average* across areas. Kids with ADHD and LD (particularly our twice exceptional kids) are more uneven. They may have 'peaks and valleys' – big differences between what they are good at and things they will have to work harder to master.

For parents of kids with ADHD, it is hard sometimes to focus on what is going well if you're being barraged with negative feedback about your child on a regular basis. Each of us has qualities and abilities to celebrate, but too often the things teachers praise are not the things kids with ADHD are naturally good at (things like sitting still and finishing work without extra help).

It is often easiest to focus on what is going wrong in our lives. Our brains are designed to look for signs of danger or problems. This is called Negativity Bias, and it keeps us out of trouble. However, if we focus too much on the negative, we get demoralized. This book is, of course, about being realistic about difficulties, but the goal is to leave you hopeful and energized. Rest assured, after we look at weaknesses, we'll show you ways to use strengths to overcome them.

WEAKNESSES

First off, we often see our children's weaknesses as permanent, as if each child came with a genetic package of abilities, talents and weaknesses. It is easy to get discouraged when you've been struggling against a challenge for a long time. Keep in mind that weaknesses depend A LOT on context. Being fast and energetic is an asset on the soccer field, a liability during fourth grade long-division worksheets. Being a daydreamer is an asset for an artist, but a liability during a spelling test. The ability to hyperfocus for hours is a real problem when a child gets 'stuck' on at task, but being able to hyperfocus is essential to success in the STEM sciences.

Remember, every weakness can be an asset, every strength a weakness – depending on what we are doing! What seems like a weakness today can actually become a critical aspect of your child's future success.

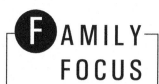

FAMILY FOCUS

"I knew he had ADHD even before he was born. He kicked me all day, all night! He went from walking to running at nine months, and was soon leaping off the coffee table. I've always been the one with 'that kid' who gets too wild, too loud, too out of control. But he's also one of the coolest kids I've ever met. Why don't people ever see that side of him?"

As parents, it is our job not to give up on a child, to write off his weaknesses as failures.

Our children's weaknesses are also not set in stone. Kids do respond well to interventions. The good news is there are many interventions that have been shown to work. Kids also mature. Their process might be slower, but it does happen. As parents it is our job not to give up on a child ... not to write off his weaknesses as failures. All of us can look back on struggles we overcame. Given that hindsight is 20-20, it is easy to see what sort of help we might have needed (or to identify those amazing times when someone believed in our potential!). Sometimes, weaknesses require the personal fortitude to wait things out for a while.

The human brain is far more 'plastic' than scientists believed in the last century. What a world it would be if nobody ever changed, grew, or matured! Your child's weaknesses are not set in stone. It is critical that your child's weaknesses not define who she is. As I've mentioned before, a weakness is not a personal failing. It is not a character flaw that will define who your child is as a person. Every person can improve, and every person will change. Just like our kids will change, we can become better parents, better advocates, and better problem solvers too. Sometimes the worst problems during childhood happen because the parent and child have the same weaknesses.

Childhood problems tend to ebb and flow. Veteran parents can tell you that what seemed like an insurmountable challenge can become just a bad memory with hard work and the passage of time. Development is on your side! Difficult times do pass – eventually.

Of course, it is unrealistic to assume that every weakness can be turned into a strength. No matter how much tutoring or special Ed or extra help we give, some things will always be areas of need. Helping our kids often depends on finding 'workarounds' or even learning to live with an imperfect situation. We cannot control the weakness, but *we can control how we choose to respond to it.*

As parents, we can help ourselves by taking time to reflect on our own strengths and weaknesses. What do we do well? For example, you might be great at tolerating noisy boys, while your spouse may get cranky because she likes order. But your spouse may be the person who dives into all the books about Special Ed law, and rocks that IEP meeting. Our self-awareness helps us make good choices for how to tackle problems.

Many situations can turn out well, or badly, depending just on how we react. We have all had the experience of a bad day turning out well in the end because of some small thing – often somebody pointing out the humor in the situation, or maybe the ice cream man appearing at just the right time. The bad day was still bad, but our perspective changed. The parent's reactions are often what sets the tone. Our sense of hope, optimism, and determination can be lifelines for our children (and our spouses!). As parents, we have a lot of power!

Of course, we can only make choices according to what we have to give. Our own strengths and weaknesses dictate what we can do on our own, and when we need to enlist help. This section is designed to help you think through your own personal resources.

Exercise #11

YOUR INVENTORY: AREAS OF WEAKNESS AND NEED

As you write your answers to the questions below try not to judge yourself, or your child, too harshly. Look carefully at the words you use, and ask yourself how accurate they really are. We all make mistakes; we all have failures. This is not a time to be beating yourself up (remember, your child needs you to teach him resilience). The point is to take an inventory of where to improve and discover where you need more support.

1. What are your family's weaknesses? What are you most concerned about?

_____

_____

_____

2. How about you and your spouse/partner/ex: when do you have trouble working as a team? What makes/made it harder for the two of you?

_____

_____

_____

3. What were your parent's greatest weaknesses, as both people and parents?

_____

_____

_____

4. When you think about yourself as a parent, what do you consider your greatest challenges?

_____

_____

_____

(continued)

EXERCISE #11 (CONTINUED)

5. What was one of the worst mistakes you made as a parent? What did you learn from that experience?

    _____

    _____

    _____

6. When have you felt the most ashamed as a parent?

    _____

    _____

7. Has there been a saddest moment for you as a parent?

    _____

    _____

8. When were you unhappy/frustrated/angry with spouse's parenting (even if you two are no longer together)?

    _____

    _____

    _____

Now think about your child's areas of need. We discussed: attentional control, behavior, emotional regulation, social skills, and executive functions.

9. What is he/she struggling with right now?

    _____

    _____

    _____

10. Which of his/her struggles has bothered you the most?

    _____

    _____

    _____

EXERCISE #11 (CONTINUED)

11. Are there any of his/her difficulties that you can relate to?

_____

_____

_____

12. Are there any difficulties you find it really hard to relate to or understand?

_____

_____

_____

13. What do you consider his/her least attractive quality? _____

_____

Remember that your child is still the same person she was before you got the diagnosis.

STRENGTHS

Time to look on the bright side!

Your child's strengths, talents, and abilities are what is going to 'pull him through.' Keep in mind that strengths often turn into careers! Plus, your family's strengths are going to get you through any tough times on the horizon as well. It is so easy to focus on the negative after your child gets a diagnosis, especially if you're feeling like you just had an emotional 'punch in the gut.' Remember that your child is still the same person she was before you got the diagnosis.

Kids with ADHD are diagnosed by a set of weaknesses. But it has been my observation that the 'flip side' of those weaknesses can be pretty fantastic. Here are some strengths I've observed among kids with ADHD:

- Spontaneity
- Playfulness
- Imagination
- Ability to hyperfocus
- Sense of fun (can lead them to be quite popular, and later, great at sales!)
- Unconventionality
- Liveliness
- Affectionateness
- Passion
- 'Outside the box' thinking and problem solving

EXERCISE #12

YOUR INVENTORY: AREAS OF STRENGTH

1. What are your family's strengths? What are you most proud of?

   _____

   _____

   _____

2. How about you and your spouse/partner/ex: what do you two do well as a team?

   _____

   _____

   _____

3. What were your own parent's greatest strengths?

   _____

   _____

   _____

4. When you think about yourself as a parent, what do you consider your best qualities and abilities?

   _____

   _____

   _____

5. When were you most proud of yourself as a parent?

   _____

   _____

6. When were you most proud of your spouse as a parent (even if you two are no longer together)?

   _____

   _____

   _____

(continued)

EXERCISE #12 (CONTINUED)

7. Now think about your child's strengths. What is he/she good at? (Being good at something doesn't necessarily mean that she's the best-ever or that he's winning awards for it).

_____

_____

_____

8. When do you feel proudest of your child?

_____

_____

9. Which of his/her accomplishments have made you most proud?

_____

_____

10. Where has your child made the most progress?

_____

_____

_____

11. What do you like best about your child?

_____

_____

12. What do other people seem to like best about your child?

_____

_____

13. Think about a time when your child overcame an obstacle? What happened?

_____

_____

EXERCISE #12 (CONTINUED)

14. What qualities do you think will help your child compensate for his difficulties? You might think of things like: people skills, energy, creativity, kindness, sense of humor, religious faith, intelligence or determination.

_____

_____

_____

_____

15. Given what your child likes and is good at, what sorts of careers might be a good fit for him/her?

_____

_____

_____

16. What good things do you wish other adults knew about your child?

_____

_____

_____

Research on resilience shows that we become resilient by learning to solve problems. The foundation to successful problem-solving is determination and grit. This is very powerful when combined with the help of a support system. The symptoms and behaviors associated with ADHD do cause extra strain – there's no way around that. But again, we choose how we will respond to that strain. Families who find ways to tackle problems together as allies are likely to look back on having a child with ADHD as transformative.

Having a common battle/challenge/mission brings people together. It creates that potent sense of 'we-ness' that deepens relationships. There's no reason to assume that having a child with a disability will hurt your marriage, damage relationships with your relatives, or mean that your child's school becomes your enemy. For some families, the strain of ADHD can be toxic, but it does not have to be! The parent's attitudes make all the difference. Many look back with a sense of pride in how they came together, and never lost hope that things could get better. Quite a few of us take pride in our battle scars.

The foundation to successful problem-solving is determination and grit. This is very powerful when combined with the help of a support system.

CHAPTER SEVEN:

TAKING CARE OF *YOU*

No two children or families are affected by ADHD in the same way. Everyone brings their own strengths to the table ... everyone has to learn to cope with weaknesses in their own way. That's why what you experience – and your Action Plan – will be different from that of every other parent who uses this book.

When we dream about having children, we never imagine having a child with a disability or a learning difference. Our daydreams are full of beautiful, perfect children who have all of our best qualities and none of our flaws.

When a child is identified as having a difference, parents grieve.

For some parents, the feeling is like a death – that child they imagined in their mind evaporates, and they must learn to love the child who is actually theirs. We can learn to love our kids, even if we don't like their behavior. The first step is accepting your child for who he is. When we understand what makes our children who they are, we can accept who they are. This *does not* mean you have to accept unwanted behaviors like hitting or jumping on the furniture. Instead, it means accepting our kids for who they are, *not who we wish they were*. Deep down we know we would never trade them for a perfect child, because they are *ours*.

Some parents feel guilt when their child has a difference.

They wonder if the child's difference happened because of something they did or failed to do. Remember, ADHD is not caused by parenting style.

Many parents feel ashamed at having had an 'imperfect' child. It can be difficult to look around at all the seemingly perfect kids out there and compare your child to the ideal you think you see. It is normal to feel jealous of other families. But remember, *every* child has some issue that parents must deal with.

It is often hard to see your child through other people's eyes.

Relatives can be particularly hurtful, even if they mean to be supportive. Many parents of children with ADHD dread school conferences and family gatherings. We may even start avoiding them because, let's face it, there's only so much we can listen to other people criticize our children.

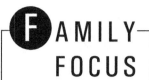

FAMILY FOCUS

"I get sick to my stomach before parent teacher conferences. I see all the other parents come out with big smiles, shaking hands with the teacher. I know they've just heard all this great stuff about their kid. I pray every time that I'll hear just one good thing . . ."

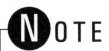

OTE

It's an opportunity to become an expert, an advocate, a better parent, and a stronger person. I always reassure 'just diagnosed' parents that they are going to discover abilities they never knew they had.

It is essential to be your child's best cheerleader.

Make sure that other people see all aspects of your child, not just how loud he is at church or her blue hair. Your child is like any other human being, he has a mix of qualities – those that are easy to love and those that give you more gray hairs.

Make sure everyone in your child's world is focused first on what is great, amazing, and special about your child. If they forget, it is your job to remind them! Take an attitude that we are going to 'build on strengths' – not focus on weaknesses.

COPING WITH THE EMOTIONAL FALLOUT OF AN ADHD DIAGNOSIS

So how are *you* doing?

This might seem beside the point – after all, this workbook is supposed to be about how to help your child. Or maybe you already rolled your eyes at hitting something 'touchy-feely.' Psychologists know that your mindset and stress level must be your immediate priority. That's because you're facing a totally new situation and to manage it, *you need to be at the top of your game.*

> *Remember: We all make our best decisions when we feel calm. We make our worst mistakes when stress clouds our thinking.*

For better or for worse, you've joined the club with those of us who have kids with a difference (yes, I'm a member too!). Raising our unique kids can be challenging at times. We often have to work harder – to dig deeper into our inner resources – than most parents do. Many days it feels unfair. Isn't just plain parenting hard enough? But just like the work, the joys can be more intense too. Many parents look back at that moment of diagnosis as a turning point in their lives. It can be a time of great meaning. But right at this moment, those lofty thoughts may not be anything like what you're actually experiencing. So let's take a look at what's going on.

THE FEELINGS KALEIDOSCOPE

The time leading up to and right after a diagnosis can be like riding a roller coaster (blindfolded – because you can't see when that next drop is coming!). If you have a spouse/partner, you two may be having very different reactions. Keep in mind that your spouse's feelings are just as legitimate as yours. There is no right or superior way to feel. You might find yourself 'taking turns' with your spouse – alternating between who feels positive or negative. One of you might be able to accept the diagnosis easily, while the other might harbor feelings of shame and anger for years.

Ignoring or stuffing your feelings down can literally make you sick. It's much healthier to just let yourself feel what you feel and recognize that when it comes to our kids, we all feel a kaleidoscope of emotions – *and all of them are totally normal.*

Whatever the feelings, it's important to understand what they are.

Ignoring or stuffing your feelings down can literally make you sick.

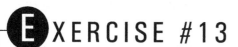 **E**XERCISE #13

KNOW YOUR FEELINGS

Circle the feelings that apply to you right now. Then have your spouse do this same exercise using a different color ink. See where the commonalties and differences are in your responses.

shocked	sad	relieved	vindicated	anxious
skeptical	hopeless	fearful	numb	overwhelmed
disappointed	protective	judged	tired	suspicious
energized	threatened	ashamed	comforted	discouraged
angry	dubious	annoyed	demoralized	combative
guilty	isolated	loving	powerless	proud
hopeful	determined			

Don't feel bad about yourself if you only circled negative emotions.
The positives will come.

If you mostly circled negatives, your emotional 'reserves' are low.
It's time to give yourself permission to take care of *you*.

Ⓕ AMILY FOCUS

I've noticed that when I tell parents they need to take time to care for *themselves*, they often argue with me. Mothers say things like: "How can I possibly take time out for me? I have three kids, my husband is out of town for work, and Marcus has a project due on forest ecosystems on Friday!" Their blood pressure shoots right up. Husbands often retort grimly that they are just fine, thank you very much.

PARENTS: GETTING ON THE SAME PAGE

If you are part of a mother and father team in your household, expect part of the adjustment process to include learning about how men vs. women handle getting a diagnosis. You will also need to be mindful of your partner or spouse's stress. Research shows that mothers and fathers deal with stress differently. If you were raised with traditional gender roles, you might find that the mother finds it easier to cry and get support. Dads raised to be tough may feel a lot of shame. Keeping shame inside is unhealthy, but many dads don't know what else to do except 'soldier on.' Most men cope with problems through action, and when no clear 'action plan' is available, frustration can build. Men often feel more comfortable expressing anger than sadness (but deep down it is all the same). Research on male and female brains has shown that women do better at handing ambiguity. Men tend to do better on tasks when there is a set of rules to follow.

If you are separated/divorced, it might be especially tough to get on the same page. If the separation was particularly acrimonious, expect the diagnosis to bring up a lot of the old conflicts. Some separated parents turn to parent coordinators or parent coaches – particularly when it comes time to make hard choices. Avoid falling into the trap of using your child's needs to settle old scores.

If you are part of a same-gender couple, this may be one of those rare times when you'll have it easier. It has been my observation that same-gender couples often have an easier time adjusting to a diagnosis. It may be that the couple's experiences with adversity actually help them cope with a child who has a difference.

FOSTERING YOUR OWN RESILIENCE

Now that we've looked at *what* you're feeling, let's look at *how* you're feeling.

For starters, your feelings about your child's differences are going to change. Some days you'll be on top of the world, ready to claim that 'Parent of the Year' award. Some days you'll look at your child with tears in your eyes, so proud of her progress you could burst. Other days you'll wonder if things will ever get easier. Other days you may be blown away by how angry you are.

Most parents of kids with differences can expect to have higher highs and lower lows in the first year.

Letting your emotional reserves get too low
is a mistake we all make.

Remember the famous advice on airplanes – put your own oxygen mask on before helping others. You know why they had to add that into the act? No doubt because parents were turning blue trying to get their kids masks on just right. Emotionally, parents of kids who have differences are often 'running on fumes.' *You can't help your child if your own emotional engine is on 'empty.'* And if you're part of a couple, putting 100% of your energy towards your child 24-7 creates even more problems than it solves.

I'm not saying you need to jump on a plane for Vegas or spend a week at the spa. There are many small but effective ways to build self-care into your day. Usually the biggest hurdle is giving ourselves permission to take the focus off doing for others, and put it back on ourselves.

When our reserves get low, we are much more likely to do things we wouldn't normally do. We find ourselves yelling at the kids or grousing at our spouse. We are irritated and quick to anger. We might also find ourselves getting too tired to keep going. Smart parents invest time in themselves. Do it as a favor to your family.

The first step in keeping your reserves from getting too low is to monitor your emotional pulse.

TAKING YOUR EMOTIONAL PULSE

Stepping back to take your own 'emotional pulse' is like checking your heart rate at the gym. It is not about being 'touchy-feely.' It is a very practical skill. Our actual pulse tells how healthy you are – whether you're ready to run a marathon or if it's time to lose a few pounds. Taking your emotional pulse helps you gauge your own available resources in the moment.

It is a skill that you'll need to practice. Once you get good at it, this skill will serve you well! When we 'step back' to examine our thoughts and feelings, we gain a sense of control over them. We also get early-warning signals about when our emotional reserves are starting to run on empty.

You can't help your child if your own emotional engine is on 'empty.'

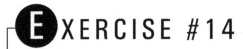

EXERCISE #14

TAKING YOUR EMOTIONAL PULSE

Sit down in a comfy chair when you have at least 2 minutes where nobody will bother you. Take a deep breath. Turn your attention inward. Now, follow the **MBA** strategy for taking your emotional pulse:

1. **MIND:** On a scale from one to ten (one being calm/peaceful and ten being overwhelmed/angry/freaking out), how are you feeling right now about your child's ADHD diagnosis?

   My emotional pulse is: 1   2   3   4   5   6   7   8   9   10

2. **BODY:** Where are you feeling this emotional intensity in your body?

   (Head, chest, abdomen?) _____

3. **ACTION:**

   • **If your emotional pulse is 5 or below,** be grateful for this moment. Keep doing what you're doing.

   • **If your emotional pulse is greater than 5,** it is time to change course. You'll need to take some time out for self-care or risk getting overwhelmed (later, we'll show you how to do that).

   • **If your emotional pulse is 7 or above,** your emotional reserves are rapidly being depleted (just like how the little yellow light pops up when your car is on Empty).

   • **If your emotional pulse is 8 or above** for days at a time, it is time to get some help to get it back down. Fortunately, there are lots of resources that can help you get your stress back down so you can do what needs to get done.

Get in the habit of taking your pulse and using the MBA strategy every day for the first week. Over time, use it whenever you have a new challenge or a tough day. Paying attention to your 'pulse' will help you identify those times when you need 'self-care.'

FOSTERING YOUR OWN RESILIENCE

Now is a critical time for self-care – right after you've received the diagnosis.

Making time for self-care improves your resilience – that ability to 'bounce back' and persevere in the face of obstacles. Building up your resilience is like packing well for a journey. If you set off tired or forget to pack the water, you may never get where you're going. Remember, you've got a long road ahead of you.

Three 'first things' to know about resilience:

- **Let yourself have a good cry** if you need to (parents cry in my office all the time – even tough people like CEOs and soldiers). You'll feel better afterward.

- ***Don't* punch a pillow.** Back in the last century, psychologists had the idea (thanks to Freud) that tension needed to be released, just like steam from an engine. Psychologists used to recommend that people express anger to 'get it out' by punching things or yelling. Current research shows that acting angry and behaving aggressively actually *makes you feel worse.*

- **Model resilience – your kids will thank you.** One of the best gifts we can give our kids is teaching them how to deal with life's ups and downs without 'going under.' So if you won't make time for self-care for your own sake, do it for your kids! If you scream at everybody or reach for the scotch when you're stressed out, *they will too.*

- **Deal with stress before it harms you.** Psychological stress and depression have consequences for our physical health. People with too much stress have depressed immune systems, low energy, gastric disturbances, and often experience chronic pain (commonly back pain and headaches).

HOW DO YOU FOSTER YOUR OWN RESILIENCE?
YOU LEARN TO USE POSITIVE COPING STRATEGIES.

A positive coping strategy heals us, making us more calm and resilient. We each need a repertoire of these strategies we can activate to bring ourselves back to a state of calm.

Positive coping tools make us healthy in body and spirit. Taking the time to write them down makes it more likely you'll actually do them! Examples might include: walking the dog, taking a nap, calling a friend, exercising, reading a trashy novel, playing a game on your phone, deep breathing, locking yourself in your room for a few minutes with a 'do not disturb' sign on the door. My clients often identify coping tools such as: watching a mediation video, taking a bath, stretching, deep breathing, praying, walking/petting the dog, stroking a cat, getting outside, looking at photos, and drinking tea.

Building up your resilience is like packing well for a journey. If you set off tired or forget to pack the water, you may never get where you're going.

It's important to make your list when you are NOT feeling frazzled.
Put your list on a little card you carry with you or on your phone – keep it handy.
Make sure to have things on the list you can do at work or in public too. That way,
when you take your 'emotional pulse' you can turn right towards doing something
healthy. This is the emotional equivalent of having fresh apples on hand when you're
hungry instead of a jumbo bag of potato chips.

ⒺXERCISE #15

IDENTIFYING YOUR OWN POSITIVE COPING TOOLS

Use the space below to make a list of 'positive coping tools' – actions you can
take that make you feel calm, refreshed, and strong.

My positive Coping Tools (have at least 5):

_____

_____

_____

_____

_____

_____

_____

_____

_____

_____

RECOGNIZE NEGATIVE COPING TRAPS

The flip side of self-care is to recognize negative coping traps. These are unhealthy things that we do to feel better (smoking, overeating, drinking). Negative coping traps make us feel good for a moment, but make the problem worse over time. We all find ourselves turning to negative coping tools because they bring such immediate relief! Eating a box of donuts brings immediate euphoria that, frankly, walking the dog just can't match. So when we are in the middle of an emotional storm, we tend to go for the negative coping traps.

Twelve-step programs have long recognized that people fall into negative coping traps when we are: hungry, angry, lonely, or tired (often called the HALT strategy to promote self-awareness). Taking our emotional pulse with the MBA strategy (remember: mind, body, action) alerts us to watch out for HALT risk factors.

How can we avoid negative coping traps so we can be the parents/spouses/ friends/employees we want to be?

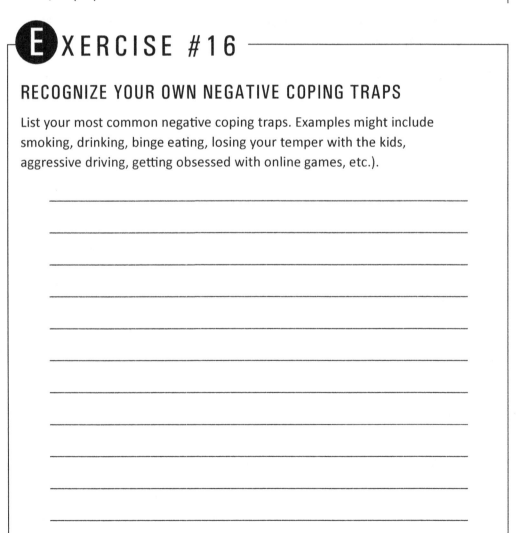

EXERCISE #16

RECOGNIZE YOUR OWN NEGATIVE COPING TRAPS

List your most common negative coping traps. Examples might include smoking, drinking, binge eating, losing your temper with the kids, aggressive driving, getting obsessed with online games, etc.).

_____

_____

_____

_____

_____

_____

_____

_____

_____

_____

LEARNING TO REFRAME

Another way to boost your resilience is to learn how to reframe your thoughts. We all have automatic thoughts that go through our heads. They can keep you from thinking clearly, and you need to think clearly if you're going to help your child. Remember, your mission is to take care of yourself so you'll have the reserves to dive in and do what needs to be done.

We often give ourselves negative messages about our parenting. Most of us hear critical voices from our childhoods as our 'inner voice.' Those phrases we heard growing up can become part of us. Thoughts like, "Can't you be more like your brother?", "You're a loser", "Don't be a crybaby", "Can't you do anything right?" make it harder to think clearly.

These are ANTs: Automatic Negative Thoughts.
Don't let them become habitual.

The good news is that we can learn to 'stomp out' ANTs. Once we recognize ANTs for what they are, we can convert them into Energizer statements. Energizer statements foster resilience. Resilience is what lets us do what needs to get done.

EXERCISE #17

TURNING ANTS INTO ENERGIZERS

Here are some common ANTs and examples of how to turn the ANTs into Energizers:

ANT example	Energizer Example
I'm a terrible parent	I'm working hard to get better
I screwed up again	I'll learn from that mistake
My kids are spoiled brats	I need a better discipline plan
This gets worse every day	This rough patch will pass
I can't take this!	I *will* get through this

Now, listen to your own thoughts. Hear what you say. Write any negative statements under the ANTs column. Then, reframe the statement as a positive Energizer.

ANT	ENERGIZER
_____	_____
_____	_____
_____	_____
_____	_____
_____	_____
_____	_____
_____	_____
_____	_____
_____	_____
_____	_____
_____	_____
_____	_____
_____	_____
_____	_____

CREATING YOUR
ADHD ACTION PLAN

CREATING YOUR ADHD ACTION PLAN

Your Action Plan will include these sections:

1. **DEALING WITH OTHERS:** Define the strategies you will use to educate others about your child and her ADHD, and deal with people who are not helping the situation.

2. **GETTING MORE INFORMATION:** Understand who can help, what information you have (and will need), what kind of testing may be helpful, and whether you will want to get an independent educational evaluation.

3. **LIFESTYLE CHANGES:** Decide on specific changes you will consider making to family life and your child's diet, routine, and other environmental factors.

4. **MEDICATION:** Understand the options available (and the potential risks and side effects) and set up a way to monitor how medications are working so you can share observations with your child's doctor most effectively.

5. **SKILLS, TRAINING AND THERAPIES:** Choose what professionals will be part of your team and what specific activities will be used to support your child and your family.

6. **EDUCATIONAL INTERVENTIONS:** Define specific steps you want to take with teachers, school counselors, tutors, etc. to support your child's academic and social success. Include when and with whom you want to schedule consultations.

Before we launch into making that Action Plan – let's consider the real goal. *Our goal is to improve the quality of life for children and ourselves!*

Remember you may need time for self-care before tackling your Action Plan.

CHAPTER EIGHT:

DEALING WITH OTHERS

For better or for worse, you are going to get very, very good at dealing with others. First things first:

DO WE TELL OUR RELATIVES?

It has been my experience that, once you are sure you have an accurate diagnosis, disclosing is the wisest course. That said, there are still probably some old fashioned or rigid relatives who are best left out of the loop. You may want to leave out the 'toxic' relatives if you can (they are probably not the ones you will trust to care for your child when you're not around anyway!).

Avoid treating the diagnosis like some family scandal. If you are frank and unemotional, your relatives hopefully will follow your lead. Be honest and positive, and emphasize what action you are taking. You don't want it to become juicy gossip. Tell your 'allies' first. Those are your best, kindest relatives who want to help (I'm hoping you have some of these). Then once they all know, they can help protect you and your child from the 'less enlightened' family members.

Be prepared for 'unenlightened' responses. When you tell someone about your child's diagnosis, you might hear a wonderful message of support and love. But odds are, you will probably hear unhelpful responses like:

- She doesn't look like she has ADHD.
- That's silly, everybody knows ADHD is over-diagnosed.
- Are you medicating him yet?
- Whatever you do, don't medicate him!
- No way, he's just being a boy. They're all like that.
- In my day, a good spanking solved problems like that.
- He's probably just gifted.
- ADHD is just a modern excuse for bad behavior.
- You know ADHD doesn't really exist, right?
- If you'd just cut out sugar/gluten/food dyes/processed foods, it would cure her.
- I knew there was something wrong with him!

The reason I include this list is because if you are ready for these comments, they're much easier to deal with.

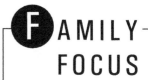

FAMILY FOCUS

"I feel sometimes like her teacher is out to get her. Just tallying up all the bad stuff to rub my nose in it. How exactly is this helping?"

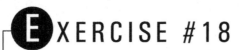

EXERCISE #18

DEALING WITH THE PERSON YOU DREAD

Everyone has that person who we dread telling the most. Take a moment to think of the *three worst possible things that person could say* (use MBA if you need to as you imagine this scene).

Now practice seeing yourself giving a really good response, calmly, from a position of strength. Remind yourself that you are the expert. Nothing anyone can say has to change how you feel, think or act! If you feel confident, their words will wash over you like a wave, and hopefully leave just as quickly.

TALKING ABOUT YOUR CHILD'S DIAGNOSIS

You want to get very good at explaining your child's diagnosis. Remember that if people don't know your child has a diagnosis, they are much more likely to label him (and you probably won't like the labels they choose!).

Keep in mind that about one out of every ten child has some sort of learning difficulty or problem that would warrant a diagnosis at any given time.

So, whom should you tell? What do you say?
There are times when you need to be proactive about disclosing the diagnosis. If your child is struggling, it is critical to share the diagnosis *before* something goes wrong. It is always easier to avoid a problem than to go back and try to fix it afterward. This means you should always tell:

- All of your child's teachers
- Adults who work with your child (coaches, tutors, babysitters)
- His physician
- Anyone who assumes responsibility for your child (e.g. the parent host of a sleepover)

When do you disclose?
Disclose whenever:

- You're going into a situation where your child's symptoms could create difficulties
- You realize that behavior expectations in a given situation are going to be very hard for your child to meet
- You are concerned your child's behavior may lead to inappropriate punishments, mistreatment, or exclusion
- You or your child might need someone's help
- Your child's safety (both emotional and physical) depends on it

You will get very good at sizing up situations for 'triggers and trouble spots' – those stumbling blocks just waiting to get in your child's way (more on this later). Still, having worked with families for over 20 years now, I know the decision to disclose your child's diagnosis is often fraught with anxiety. If, in the previous chapter, you identified a lot of feelings of shame or embarrassment over having a child with a difference, you'll need more support on your journey.

All parents fear that their child will be judged, rejected, underestimated or excluded. *Those fears are legitimate.* We all know that stigma around mental health disorders is real – there's no sugar coating it. Keep in mind that about one out of every ten children has some sort of learning difficulty or problem that would warrant a diagnosis at any given time. Learning and mental health problems are more common than most people realize! Stigma arises from ignorance. Fighting that stigma is the reason that books like these exist. The more people who disclose their mental health diagnoses (demand fair treatment) the better we can fight the stigma. If we act like our child's diagnosis is a shameful secret, other people will too. Every time you disclose, you teach people how to think about your child.

It has been my experience that when families resisted disclosing the diagnosis, other people still noticed the child's difficulties. The difference is that they tried to understand what they were seeing by labeling the child (and often, the parents).

IT IS GENERALLY BETTER TO BE PROACTIVE RATHER THAN REACTIVE

Again, don't wait for something to go wrong! For example, giving a teacher or a karate instructor a quick 'heads up' about what your child needs to be successful can save everyone a lot of frustration. It can also help others be more patient with your child, and thus less likely to judge or punish. It is generally essential to disclose if you are depending on an adult to keep your child safe, such as on a field trip or sleepover.

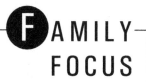

FAMILY FOCUS

"My mother-in-law is driving me crazy. She's really old school and doesn't believe in ADHD. She's convinced that I'm not strict enough. To make it worse, she's always comparing my kids to my sister's perfect children. This year at Thanksgiving I overheard her complaining to the relatives about all the bad stuff my kids do."

EXERCISE #19

DECIDING WHO NEEDS TO KNOW

Be proactive! Make a list of situations your child is likely to encounter in the next year. For which does it make sense to tell the other adults about your child's diagnosis? Here are samples to consider:

- A new classroom or school
- A birthday party
- Eating in a fancy restaurant
- A sleepover
- Visiting friends/relatives who have no kids and lots of antiques

- Religious services (weddings, bar/ bat mitzvah, first communion)
- Joining a new team/club
- School field trips
- Vacations/travel

PRACTICAL TIPS ON DISCLOSURE

It's often in your child's best interest to disclose his difference to others.
This allows people to accommodate him as well as to treat him with compassion. After all, ADHD is nothing to be ashamed of!

If you're having a tough time with disclosure, don't 'go it alone.'
Intellectually, you know that ADHD is nothing to be ashamed of — no more than diabetes or a broken arm. That said, you may be deeply troubled at having an 'imperfect' child (if a perfect child exists, I have yet to see it). This is especially so if your family of origin is perfectionistic or intolerant of differences. If in the previous section you identified a lot of feelings of grief or shame, your 'self-care' should include finding a professional to help heal. Licensed or certified psychologists, counselors, or social workers are great resources.

Remember that ADHD is a 'hidden disability.'
The advantage is that people won't think of your child as different. The disadvantage is that people are going to assume your child is just a regular kid. As a result, they will often assume that your child's behavior is something he or she can choose and control. *Most adults know very little about what a child can or cannot do at a given age. They know even less about what **your** child can and cannot do.* For example, a child with ADHD may just have an impulse to shove something, act on it, and be shocked when the desk falls over onto a classmate's foot. Did the child in this example intend to hurt his classmate? No. Will that keep the principal from suspending him? Not unless that principal understands that child has ADHD.

Never assume people, even professionals, have accurate information.
Having degrees and titles does not necessarily mean a person knows more about what is right for your child than you do!

Having degrees and titles does not necessarily mean a person knows more about what is right for your child than you do!

CREATE YOUR 'ADVOCACY ELEVATOR PITCH'

You'll need to get good at explaining who your child is and what he needs – clearly and succinctly. In business, we call this making an 'elevator pitch.' This means it has to be quick enough that you could 'pitch' your company's services in the time allotted in a typical elevator trip. Elevator pitches cut to the chase of what matters most. They also serve to create a framework in other people's minds, which lets you get a conversation, meeting or appointment with a new professional starting off on the right track.

An elevator pitch should emphasize strengths, areas of need, diagnosis, and the 'zinger' – something special about your child that makes her memorable.

Example One: Jake

Our son Jake is a fourth grader at Riverbend Elementary School. Jake has been found to be intellectually gifted, but his symptoms of hyperactivity get in his way of achieving at his ability level. He has also struggled to make and keep new friends. Jake was recently diagnosed with ADHD – Hyperactive Type. We have found that Jake does best when he can move a lot and study science. This year he's been ecstatic about his teacher's Chesapeake Bay ecosystems project.

Example Two: Maria

My daughter Maria is a 6th grader at St. Vincent's Catholic School. Maria is exceptionally kind. She wants very much to please her teachers. Her symptoms of distractibility and weak organizational skills have become a big obstacle after she transitioned to the middle school program. Right now, she might fail English. When she was in 3rd grade, she was diagnosed with ADHD, Inattentive Type. We have found that she does her best in small classes with a lot of individual prompting. She has always loved art. This year, her main interest has become drawing fantasy characters.

Elevator pitches cut to the chase of what matters most. They also serve to create a framework in other people's minds, which lets you get a conversation, meeting or appointment with a new professional starting off on the right track.

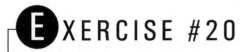

CREATE YOUR OWN ADHD ELEVATOR PITCH

Imagine you are talking to a new teacher about your child. Try to create an Elevator Pitch that introduces your child in a positive way, mentions the type of ADHD diagnosis and key issues, your concerns, what works and an example of something your child loves or where he shines. Keep honing your pitch until you have it down to about 45-60 seconds.

_____

_____

_____

_____

_____

_____

_____

_____

_____

_____

_____

_____

_____

_____

_____

_____

_____

_____

_____

_____

DEALING WITH OTHER PEOPLE

In your journey of raising a child with a difference, you are going to encounter wonderful people who will go the extra mile to help your child.
Unfortunately, you will also have to deal with all the rest.

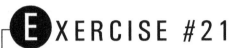

EXERCISE #21

IDENTIFYING THE UN-SUPER HEROES IN YOUR CHILD'S LIFE

Circle the 'characters' in your child's life:

the ignorant	the bigoted	the judger
the snob	the condescender	the perfect parent
the know-it-all	the rigid	the clueless
the well meaning	the mean	the disinterested
the biased	the saboteur	the intolerant
the over-reactor	the pessimist	the dismissive
the toxic	the overly-optimistic	the control freak
the misinformed	the passive aggressive	

But wait, aren't labels bad?

Remember, if you see people as labels, you give up on them. Don't! You are going to need all the allies you can get, especially if your family has to get through the next five years of elementary school with these people.

Look at the Un-Super Hero labels you circled and pick three that made you think of people in your life. For each one, consider if this is a person you could turn from an obstacle into an ally. While 'the mean' or 'the toxic' might never change, you can often make good progress with the people who have no idea they are making your life harder (e.g. the ignorant, the over-reactor).

Now, instead of deciding that these people are roadblocks, start thinking about how you can work with them.

Everybody acts the way they do for two main reasons: their behavior gets them something they want; their behavior helps them avoid something uncomfortable (remember the ABCs of behavior?). For example:

- 'The Rigid' person wants order and predictability because they fear loss of control (often the same as the 'over-reactor').

- 'The Saboteur' may need to be proven right so she can avoid looking stupid at all costs.

- 'The Clueless' may want to find simple solutions so he doesn't have to take on a lot of extra work.

Once you figure out what is motivating the behavior (the antecedents) it's easier to relate to these difficult people, and easier for you to work with them as part of a team.

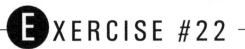 **XERCISE #22**

STRATEGIES FOR TURNING UN-SUPER HEROES INTO ALLIES

Fill in this chart to help think of your strategies. I did two examples for you.

The Un-Superhero	What does he want?	What does he fear?	Ideas for turning him into an ally
the misinformed	to be an expert	looking ignorant	share new research/ask for his expertise
the judger	to feel good about herself	looking incompetent	ask for her advice/opinion

HELPING OTHERS WORK WITH YOUR CHILD

Remember when you wrote about what engaged your child's attention? For building on strengths, let's go more in-depth. Remember that kids with ADHD can pay attention if their attentional system is engaged.

To help professionals understand how to work with your child, you need to be able to explain how to engage him. Take the time to think it through. You may wish to use these questions to write a little letter of introduction or Frequently Asked Questions list for professionals who will be working with your child.

Use the following questions to guide you. Even if you don't write the answers out to give to people, you should get to the point where you can provide this information (the question answers) without having to stop and think. Practicing your answers will make you more confident and assertive – good qualities to have when advocating for your child!

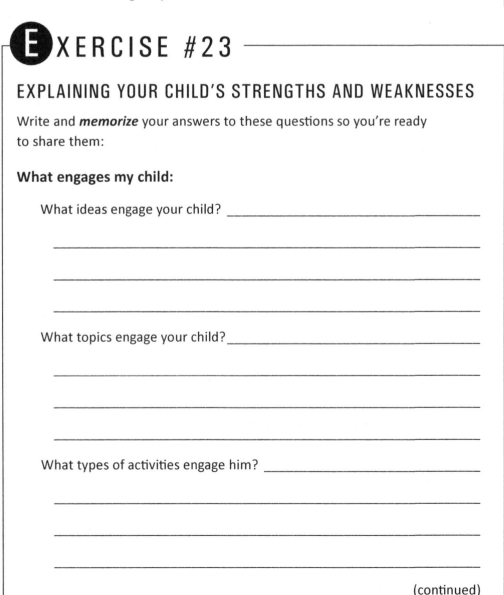

EXERCISE #23

EXPLAINING YOUR CHILD'S STRENGTHS AND WEAKNESSES

Write and *memorize* your answers to these questions so you're ready to share them:

What engages my child:

What ideas engage your child? _____

_____

_____

What topics engage your child?_____

_____

_____

What types of activities engage him? _____

_____

_____

(continued)

EXERCISE #23 (CONTINUED)

What types of environments engage her?_____

_____

_____

_____

When is he at his best? _____

_____

_____

_____

What qualities in an adult does he respond best to? _____

_____

_____

_____

What kinds of peers help her be at her best? _____

_____

_____

_____

How often does he need a break from a preferred/engaging activity? ____

_____

_____

_____

What makes life harder for your child?

What ideas 'turn-off' your child?_____

_____

_____

_____

EXERCISE #23 (CONTINUED)

What topics do not interest him? _____

_____

_____

_____

What activities does he dislike? _____

_____

_____

_____

What types of activities does he find frustrating or boring? _____

_____

_____

What environments trigger behavior or focus difficulties? _____

_____

_____

When is he at his worst? _____

_____

_____

What qualities in an adult throw him off? _____

_____

_____

What kind of peers does he find it hardest to be with? _____

_____

_____

How often does he need a break from a non-preferred activity? _____

_____

_____

CHAPTER NINE:

GETTING MORE INFORMATION

START BY KEEPING TRACK

Parents often forget the details of that first diagnosis. The history of your child's issues is important. Take a few minutes to capture the following information:

1. When was my child diagnosed? _____

2. Who made the initial referral? _____

3. Who did the first diagnosis? _____

4. What were my top three concerns at the time?

   _____

   _____

   _____

5. What information was gathered to determine the diagnosis? If you received a report, the types of data collected should be listed, such as names of tests or who was interviewed.

   _____

   _____

   _____

6. Think for a moment about what led you to have your child evaluated for ADHD. Was it only because of concerns listed on the DSM list, or did you have other concerns? What else first concerned you or other people in your child's life?

   _____

   _____

   _____

The history of your child's issues is important. Take a few minutes to capture the following information.

***Your Action Plan needs to define who can help you,
what information you have and will need,
and what kind of testing may be helpful.***

FOR STARTERS, YOU MIGHT WANT TO HAVE NEUROPSYCHOLOGICAL TESTING FOR YOUR CHILD

Remember that about half of all kids with ADHD also have learning disabilities. Children with ADHD are at higher risk for emotional difficulties, including poor self-concept, anxiety and depression. You may just want to get a sense of what your child is capable of, or how she learns best.

Parents often wonder how to 'shop' for psychological testing.
Testing is hard to shop for, mostly because you've never bought it before. It's not like a car, where we have a sense of what is a good car, and can take one for a test drive if we like.

Look for a licensed psychologist or licensed clinical psychologist (the specific title varies from state to state). You may also find a neuropsychologist (who will be a licensed psychologist with advanced training in how the brain functions). Only a licensed psychologist can call him or herself a psychologist. Other professionals can call themselves therapists, counselors, or education/ behavior specialists, but no one else can say they are a psychologist. The professional license means that the psychologist has extensive training, graduated from doctoral program (PhD, PsyD, or Ed.D.), completed a clinical internship/residency and, most of the time, also did a post-doctoral year or two. Finally, the psychologist has proven him/herself by passing national and state examinations. The license also means that the State Board of Health Professions is there to protect the public from any psychologist's failure to live up to professional standards.

Set up parameters.
Define how much you can comfortably spend on testing, how far you can travel, and how soon you need results.

Ask for referrals.

The best people to ask are professionals who use psychological testing reports to do their jobs, including:

- Special education advocates

- Special education teachers

- Special education attorneys

- Pediatricians can be hit or miss. Some do a lot of collaborating with psychologists, while others almost never do. Not all pediatricians have a great deal of experience with the special education system. A report that looks great from a medical standpoint might be almost useless in an IEP meeting.

- Advocacy groups are a good choice since they have relationships with local psychologists and have a large member base you can consult.

- Beware of the internet! Online reviews are great for picking out the best thin crust pizza or coffee maker. People who post information about their children's psychological evaluation may not be objective, and are not necessarily able to give you good advice about your own situation. Message boards can also be full of fake reviews as well, so a 'five star' rating may just mean the psychologist has a lot of aunts with extra time on their hands.

TESTING THROUGH THE SCHOOL SYSTEM

You may decide to get your testing through the school system. Testing will be done either by a Licensed Psychologist or a School Psychologist (who may have a doctoral degree or a master's degree).

The advantage of school testing is that it is free.

It also happens during the school day so you don't have to take off work. You can also be assured your child is in a familiar setting (assuming he feels positively about school, that's a plus). Sometimes it is an advantage to have your child work with a familiar adult, sometimes a set of fresh eyes is warranted.

The downside is that the school staff's task is not actually to diagnose ADHD.

Their task is to screen for which children meet eligibility criteria for special education services. Those are two different tasks. School psychologists are not supposed to make a diagnosis – that decision is shared by the school's Multidisciplinary Team of professionals. Since their task is identifying which children qualify for special education, the school system generally does not provide as in-depth testing as a private psychologist or hospital.

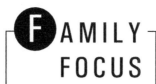

FAMILY FOCUS

"These school meetings can really get you down. We are experienced now, and we know our rights. I've become quite an expert on Special Ed law, because I've had to. When we were just starting out, we used to just take their word for it. Then I'd make a mad dash for the car so I could cry it out. We've learned how to play this game – when to push and how!"

The testing at schools is piecemeal – split up among professionals.
The psychologist does the IQ test, the special educator does the academic testing, and often a social worker interviews the family. This lack of continuity can be problematic when everyone is trying to figure out exactly what is going on with the child. If your child's issues are fairly straightforward, and there is a clear educational impact of his or her disability, school testing can be a good choice.

TESTING IN A MEDICAL SETTING OR COMMUNITY MENTAL HEALTH CENTER

You may want to have your child assessed at a pediatric hospital. Large cities often have medical centers where they do a lot of evaluations. If your child is atypical in some way – perhaps was born before 32 weeks' gestation, has had significant head injuries, or has a rare genetic difference – a hospital is a good choice. The other good thing about a hospital is that they will take your insurance, whatever type you have.

You may also select a community mental health center. This might be run by the county or state, or might be part of a nonprofit agency. Some are managed by religious organizations such as Catholic Charities or Jewish Social Services. It does not matter if you are not of that faith.

The downside is often the quality of the experience.
Medical centers can be intimidating for children. Little ones may worry about getting shots or medical procedures. There are sometimes strange smells, or sick or injured children in the area. Your child may also have to finish the testing in one day's marathon appointment. Community mental health centers are not known for being luxurious, but they should be easy to get to from public transportation.

If you are having the testing done in a teaching hospital or community mental health center, you may have a student or resident doing the testing. If your child can be difficult to handle, a student with less experience may have trouble managing his or her behavior. Learning to get a child through testing, and to give his best effort, is a skill that takes years to develop. If you can, go with a more experienced clinician (preferably one who has their own kids – no training in the world is more educational than having your own children).

If the hospital is not a teaching hospital, your child may be tested by a 'technician' or person who has yet to earn a psychologist's license. This person administers and scores tests under supervision of a psychologist. He or she may draft the report for the psychologist and both will sign it. You will want to know this person's qualifications.

The other good thing about a hospital is that they will take your insurance, whatever type you have.

While some students and technicians do a good job, you may have to sacrifice having your child actually work with a psychologist. Instead of getting to know one person, the child might be passed from person to person, so that each trainee can get the practice she needs. As a result, hospital reports are often very impersonal. Psychologists in medical centers often save time from their busy schedules by dictating their reports instead of writing them by hand, so they can be somewhat boilerplate (sometimes literally just a template where your child's name and scores get dictated into the form). Community centers generally do not have sophisticated dictation systems, and so the report is likely to be more personal.

Most importantly, you may be on a waiting list for as long as six months. You may also be waiting for your report for quite some time, particularly if a student is the one preparing it under supervision. Teaching someone to write a report takes time, and supervising psychologists may take a long time to finally sign off on the finished product.

TESTING IN A PRIVATE PRACTICE

The benefits of choosing private practice are that, since you are a paying client, you have more control over your experience. The office should be less medical, and hopefully welcoming to children. Wait lists should be shorter, and you should (ideally) know how long you have to wait to get your report.

Private practice focuses attention and time on your child.
The psychologist should be able to be flexible about how many days it takes to complete the testing. The psychologist ideally has the ability to take his or her time to understand your child fully. Psychologists in private practice often have a wider variety of tests than a school (though perhaps less than a medical center). *This means they can select the tests that are best suited to answering your questions, not just using the ones the school system has approved.*

There are downsides to private testing, too.
Private testing is often not seen as a 'medical necessity' by your insurance company. Even if they agree in advance to pay a portion of your expenses (preauthorization), they may not follow through with their commitment. You may be paying the bulk of the fees out of pocket. Make sure you are ready to accept the bill if your insurance company refuses to help.

Dealing with insurance can be difficult.
Most claims are rejected the first time. Insurance companies pay psychologists such small amounts (if they actually pay at all), that it is difficult for psychologists who test to work with insurance companies. Some who do accept insurance have to make ends meet by using technicians or doing shorter reports. Again, this does not mean that they cannot do very good work, but it is good to choose your psychologist knowing what factors to consider.

Psychologists in private practice often have a wider variety of tests than a school (though perhaps less than a medical center). **This means they can select the tests that are best suited to answering your questions, not just using the ones the school system has approved.**

Psychological testing is expensive.

This is because, done properly, psychological testing takes many hours of work and considerable skill. A psychologist must also regularly invest considerable money in testing supplies and continuing education to stay current.

If you engage a 'fee for service' or 'out of network' psychologist, expect that you may end up being responsible for the whole bill. Do not count on your insurance company covering more than a small part, if they reimburse you at all.

Psychologists recognize that the costs are a barrier to many families. Many offer payment plans or do some pro bono or reduced fee work. Don't be afraid to ask! Believe me, psychologists in private practice are accustomed to talking with clients about how to manage fees.

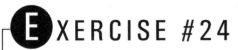

EXERCISE #24

'SHOPPING' FOR A PRIVATE PSYCHOLOGIST

When shopping for a private psychologist, make sure you have the following questions answered before you put down your deposit:

1. Will the psychologist actually do the testing? If not, how many people will my child work with? What are the qualifications of those people? Are any students?

2. After testing, when can I expect my report?

3. Will you consult with my child's team (educators, pediatricians, and psychiatrist)?

4. Can you do an observation at school if I have behavior concerns?

5. Do you have expertise in testing children with similar concerns as my child?

6. Can you break the testing up over more than one day if my child becomes tired or frustrated?

7. Do I have to stay in the office the whole time that my child is there?

INDEPENDENT EDUCATIONAL EVALUATIONS

If you have had testing through the public school system and disagree with the results, you can apply for an Independent Educational Evaluation (IEE). You'll need to make a request to the office of special education for your county in writing. If your request is granted, the school system will pay for your child to have private testing. Do not assume your request has been granted until you have a commitment from the school system in writing.

Any licensed psychologist can perform the testing. You might want to select one from the approved list the county provides. These people are experienced in conducting IEEs, and will be able to offer guidance to you in navigating the special education appeals process.

For your Action Plan: decide if you need more testing. If yes, start investigating the options that seem right for your family.

CHAPTER TEN:

LIFESTYLE CHANGES

Lifestyle changes generally cost nothing and have only positive side effects!

EXERCISE

Research strongly supports the power of exercise for improving attention and executive functioning. Researcher John Ratey has been a champion of this cause, founding the Sparking Life movement. Exercise also improves and stabilizes mood – stimulating the brain to produce 'feel good' dopamine and norepinephrine.

> **In some studies, exercise surpasses antidepressants in its effectiveness.**

If you have a child with ADHD, one of the most important things you can do to treat the symptoms is get your child exercising hard and often.

Exercise improves and stabilizes mood stimulating the brain to produce 'feel good' dopamine and norepinephrine.

SLEEP

Sleep deprivation looks a lot like ADHD. When we are sleep deprived, we are inattentive, have poor working memory, and are irritable. Unfortunately, just like a person who has had too much to drink, we don't recognize how truly impaired we are.

The American Academy of Pediatrics and other public health organizations have guides for how much your child should sleep at his age. It would be hard to overestimate how sleep deprived our teenagers are.

Good sleep habits include:

- No screens for at least 30 minutes before sleep
- Use the bed only for sleeping
- Have the child sleep in his or her own bed (not yours, not with you sleeping in his bed with him)
- Have a regular bed and wake up time

Unfortunately, the early promise of 'cure all' diets has not stood up to the test of scientific scrutiny.

DIET

Much has been written about diet and its impact on ADHD. Unfortunately, the early promise of 'cure all' diets has not stood up to the test of scientific scrutiny.

For most children, eating organic food or cutting out gluten will probably not do much to change their symptoms. Some children have sensitivities to food dyes, but most do not.

It is a myth that sugar causes hyperactivity (I promise; this has been tested). That said, I cannot stress enough the importance of a nutritious diet that keeps blood sugar reasonably stable.

Our kids with ADHD need every advantage we can give them. Diets with fruits, vegetables and lean protein (with the occasional Happy Meal here and there) help us be at our best.

CHAPTER ELEVEN:

MEDICATION

Medication has been used to treat ADHD since the early part of the 1900s. Stimulants have emerged as the most reliable medical treatment for reducing symptoms of ADHD.

Why are stimulants effective?
Because they correct the under-arousal of the brain by increasing the availability of dopamine and norepinephrine (but remember, exercise does this too!).

Stimulants are among the safest prescription drugs prescribed for children – even safer than some over-the-counter medications. If a child truly has ADHD, it is likely that stimulants could help reduce his symptoms.

A prescription is required.
Stimulants and stimulant alternatives (atomoxetine) can be prescribed by a pediatrician. If your child has issues in addition to ADHD that make prescribing harder, you may want to ask for a referral to a pediatric psychiatrist.

Only a physician or psychiatrist can prescribe medications.
While psychologists can provide information and education about medications, in most states, only a physician can prescribe them. Your psychologist should have recommendations for you about choosing to explore medication or not, but you will need your child's doctor or psychiatrist to write the actual prescription.

It is important to work with a reputable medical professional.
'Alternative' providers may not have appropriate credentials to treat your child. They may not be licensed (a license is a good thing because it means a Board is watching over licensed professionals).

Be extremely cautious with supplements.
Some parents want to try 'natural' solutions like herbs and supplements. In this country, supplements are not regulated like medications or food. Studies have shown that the contents of supplements may have unhealthy compounds, or may not contain significant amounts of the ingredients you intended to purchase. While it sounds appealing to take a 'natural' approach, be aware that many of the supplements have never been appropriately tested on children. Mixing supplements (and I've seen kids taking as many as eight at one time) can be dangerous.

FAMILY FOCUS

"For years I thought my daughter was lazy. I grew up in a household where I had to pitch in, and I've been working since I was 14 years old. Work ethic is very important to me, so I admit I was ashamed of her, and really disappointed. It was such a turnaround when we started the medication. I was so anti-meds I held out for over a year. Finally, I gave in. My health plan changed so we could get a better pediatrician. He convinced me to let him try to help with meds. It was like the fog lifted and the real Rachel finally shone through."

Remember, if something is strong enough to help your child, it is strong enough to hurt your child.

Some herbal remedies have been researched (e.g. St. John's Wort). If you want to use alternative treatments, do so only under the guidance of your physician. Remember, if something is strong enough to help your child, it is strong enough to hurt your child.

My take? If you want a proven natural approach, exercise is your best bet.

Only *you* make the decision about medication for your child. It is not the place of teachers, principals, daycare providers, babysitters, or any other non-licensed person to encourage you to get your child medicated. Schools cannot insist that your child take medication.

SHOULD I EXPLORE MEDICATION FOR MY CHILD?

Many people have strong feelings about medication. Take a moment to think about yours. Are you open to the idea of medicating your child?

About three out of every four kids will benefit from a given stimulant. However, medication is just one tool to consider for your Action Plan, same as any other. The truth is that medication helps a lot of people. Medication helps children 'put on the brakes' so they can focus and control impulses. Your physician's goal in prescribing medication is to find the right medication and dose to hit the 'sweet spot' – the point where your child benefits, but side effects are still tolerable.

The most important factors to consider are related to quality of life. If your child's problems are very mild, and his behavior pretty easy to manage, medication may not be your first choice. My bias is that if other interventions seem to have more promise, medication should be deferred. However, you don't want to let problems spiral out of control without considering all options open to you. As I said, medications help a lot of children. As a starting point for making your own decision, I encourage you to look at the pros and cons.

First, the pros of medication:

1. Stimulants are relatively quite safe

2. Stimulants work for most children

3. Stimulants work fast (unlike all the other interventions)

4. Stimulants can be used or not used whenever you want

Cons of medication:

1. Stimulants cause some side effects

2. It can take some time and experimentation to find a medicine that helps your own unique child without causing too many side effects

3. It can be a hassle to manage all the details of maintaining and filling prescriptions and making sure your child takes the medication on the right schedule

4. Stimulants can tempt us to stop trying other forms of support

What's the most important factor to consider?

For me, the consideration that really tips the scales is: how much are the symptoms of ADHD interfering with your family's quality of life? If your child's ADHD is having a detrimental impact on his/her quality of life, or on the family's quality of life, medication might be worth exploring.

Here are some good reasons to consider medication:

1. Your child cannot learn and make progress in school because of her symptoms

2. Your child feels bad about him or herself

3. Your child's behavior prevents him from making and keeping friends

4. Your child's behavior is chaotic or dangerous (particularly if siblings are at risk)

5. Your child hates school or tries to refuse to go

6. Your child's anxiety or irritability concern you

7. Your child's symptoms make life overly stressful to manage across settings

And now, 'not so good' reasons to consider medication:

1. The school is pressuring you into it

2. It is the only treatment your insurance company will cover

3. You or your spouse don't like the idea of therapy

4. You want your child to have every advantage so he can go to an Ivy League college

5. It requires the least effort compared to other interventions

124

CHAPTER TWELVE:

SKILLS, TRAINING AND THERAPIES

Remember medication reduces symptoms, but it cannot teach skills. Effective coping skills are powerful tools your child can use his whole life long. For this piece of your Action Plan, we need to look at ways to help your child develop these skills.

MANY PARENTS (ESPECIALLY FATHERS) RESIST THE IDEA OF SEEKING THERAPY

Parents are often tempted to try to avoid therapy.
Part of this is a response to stigma, or wondering what relatives will think. We also have the idea in our culture that we should not need help parenting our kids.

Somehow we Americans have the idea that you should be a 'do it yourselfer' with the most difficult job we will ever do – raising children.
Parenting books are a great place to start, and you can check my Resources Guide for good ones (page 147), but they are not the same as having a professional's help. Anyone who has learned a complex skill (playing a musical instrument, improving your golf game) can attest to how much faster and richer the process is if you're in the hands of a great coach. Think of a therapist as your coach.

Some seem to think that good parents do not need therapy for their kids.
The myth is that only bad parents need therapy for their kids. This is not the case. Getting therapy for your child is no more a failure than taking her for any other doctor's appointment. Nobody gets upset about the idea of hiring a tutor or coach, or having someone else cut your child's hair. A therapist is just another one of the many professionals who will help your child in his life.

MAKING PSYCHOTHERAPY PART OF THE PLAN

We now know that brains can change how they function throughout the lifespan. Psychotherapy (just like good teaching) rewires the brain.

Psychotherapy takes advantage of our brain's wonderful abilities to learn and change. This adaptive capacity is called neuroplasticity. Psychotherapy is an evidence-based treatment with no side effects. Psychotherapy has also been shown to have longer lasting effects than medication alone. It promotes resilience, so that children become stronger in the face of future obstacles, too.

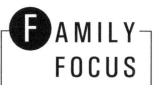

FAMILY FOCUS

"All my life I've coped with chaos. My ADHD has been a drag on me as long as I can remember. I hated school and nobody there seemed to like me much. As an adult, I've barely held it together. I miss deadlines, forget bills, never remember to change the oil in my car. It was ok when it was just me, but once I had kids it was like we were on a speeding bus with no breaks. I had to get help for myself before I could help them. They needed me to be a grown up. So I got treatment."

No license means no guarantee of training, and nobody watching out to make sure they provide quality care.

WHAT KIND OF THERAPIST IS RIGHT FOR YOUR CHILD – AND FAMILY?

There are many types of therapists. Again, pick someone who is professionally licensed! Here are the titles of licensed mental health providers:

- Psychologist
- Psychiatrist
- Licensed Professional Counselor
- Licensed Clinical Social Worker
- Marriage and Family Therapist
- Art Therapist
- Pastoral Counselor (requires a license in most states)

ADD OTHER MEMBERS TO YOUR TEAM, BUT *CHECK THEIR CREDENTIALS!*

Tutors, coaches, consultants, advocates and 'specialists' can also help your child and family develop important skills for coping with ADHD. However, proceed with caution. They may indeed be certified, qualified individuals, but check their credentials to make sure. If they hold a certificate of some kind, take the time to see how much training it actually takes to get that certificate. For example: since the title 'coach' is not regulated, anyone can use it. *Remember, no license means no guarantee of training, and nobody watching out to make sure they provide quality care.*

EXPLORING THE RIGHT KIND OF THERAPY FOR YOUR CHILD AND FAMILY

There are also many types of psychotherapy. Therapy that has been shown to be most effective for children with ADHD includes:

- Cognitive Behavior Therapy
- Behavior Therapy
- Parent Management Training
- Parent Coaching/Parent Behavior Therapy

These forms of therapy have something in common. They are goal-oriented and structured.

They focus on teaching parents and children with ADHD new skills. Most importantly, they have been well researched and found to be effective.

Parents should avoid forms of therapy that are *not* goal-oriented.
Children with ADHD desperately need help with the specific problems that their symptoms and behaviors create. They need therapy to target these high priorities!

GETTING TOP VALUE FOR YOUR INVESTMENT IN THERAPY

Therapy gets a 'bad rap' for being expensive and ineffective. This is a shame, because the evidence shows that good therapy is highly beneficial, both for current problems and for developing resilience that lasts a lifetime. Unlike medication, therapy has no side effects. If you know how to 'shop' for good therapy, you can expect it to make life better. You can avoid the types of therapies that are *unlikely* to help your child by doing your homework.

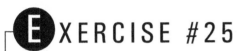

EXERCISE #25

HOW TO INTERVIEW POTENTIAL MEMBERS OF YOUR CHILD'S SUPPORT TEAM

1. **There are different types of therapy and approaches to skill-building.**
   Do your homework by asking the therapist the following questions:

   - Do you frequently treat children with ADHD?
   - Do you generally treat children my child's age?
   - What form of therapy do you do?
   - How involved will we, the parents, be in the treatment?
   - Will you be able to provide us with parent coaching?

2. **When you speak to the therapist, ask them to describe how they might work with a child like yours.**
   You may need to pay for their time to have this conversation. Investing in taking the therapist for a 'test drive' is far cheaper than paying for ineffective treatment for months (or even years)!

3. **Avoid the therapist who cannot articulate a plan for your child's treatment.**

4. **Avoid therapists who use words like 'non-directive' or 'expressive.'**
   These people often do good work, but do not offer the most effective treatments for typical problems of ADHD. You're looking for someone who knows how to use Cognitive Behavioral Therapy (CBT) with children. Children as young as three can benefit from CBT.

Parents are the key to effective therapy! Without parents helping the child change in the 'real world,' it is unlikely that the child will make much progress.

TAKING AN ACTIVE ROLE IN YOUR CHILD'S CARE

Make sure that you (and your spouse or co-parent) will be active participants in your child's care. The younger the child, the more the treatment should involve parent coaching.

You should be learning: what your child is working on, learning skills for supporting his progress, and perhaps even learning to use a behavior plan. Parents are the key to effective therapy! Without parents helping the child change in the 'real world,' it is unlikely that the child will make much progress.

EFFECTIVE, EVIDENCE-BASED THERAPY

What effective, evidence-based therapy teaches children:

- How to recognize, name, and cope with strong feelings
- How to make wise choices
- Better social skills
- 'Positive Opposite' behaviors to replace undesirable behaviors
- Self-control
- Mindfulness
- Meditation/guided visualization/relaxation techniques

What effective, evidence-based therapy teaches parents:

- How to spot children's 'triggers' (antecedents)
- How to help children cope with strong feelings (emotion coaching)
- Specific problem-solving strategies (e.g. Ross Greene's 'Collaborative Problem Solving Approach')
- How to increase levels of desirable behaviors
- How to reduce or get rid of undesirable behaviors
- How to avoid inadvertently encouraging undesirable behaviors
- How to implement effective consequences
- How to cope with their own strong emotions

SHOULD YOU CONSIDER GROUP THERAPY?

Typically, group therapy programs for kids teach skills like social skills, coping skills, mindfulness/relaxation, or ways to solve everyday problems.

Many children, especially teens, like the energy of a group. Teenagers may find it easier to talk about their problems with other teens while the group leader facilitates. Younger children can practice important skills like learning to share toys or use good manners.

The upside:
Group therapy can also be cheaper!

The downside:
First, there are usually waiting lists. Second, it can be tough to find a group that is a good 'fit' for your child. Before you enter a group, the leader should do an intake session with you to make sure your child and the group will be compatible.

A WORD ABOUT BRAIN TRAINING SOFTWARE

There has been a lot of 'buzz' about brain training software. Some practices offer therapeutic software programs designed to improve working memory and attention. You may also hear ads for companies that sell software, apps, or web-based services that claim to improve memory, attention, and problem-solving skills.

At this time, the 'jury is still out' as to whether these products can actually improve a person's real-world functioning. These software programs may simply help people get better at doing the tasks in the software, without having any permanent impact on daily life. These are interventions that might help, but we don't know that they will.

In my professional opinion, it is too early to tell (based on current research) if it is worth taking time and money away from other interventions that have been shown to be effective. My own recommendation is that you have your child spend his or her time exercising instead of spending more time sitting still with a screen. There is a very solid research base showing the impact of exercise!

At this time, the 'jury is still out' as to whether these products can actually improve a person's real-world functioning.

CHAPTER THIRTEEN:

EDUCATIONAL INTERVENTIONS

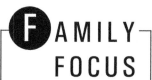

Your child spends about six hours in school every day. Effective interventions for ADHD have to target what happens at school, too. Small changes to the learning environment can come with a big payoff!

When most people think of school interventions, they think of special education. Your child may not actually need special education. Sometimes changes like a new school that has more recess and PE every day can be just what the doctor ordered.

What can be done outside of special education:
- A new school that allows for more movement or a more active, 'hands-on' educational experience
- Hiring a tutor or ADHD Coach to support your child
- Using assistive technology (word processors, graphic organizers, and organizational software)

SPECIAL EDUCATION INTERVENTIONS _____

It is beyond the scope of this book to go into great detail about special education, but I will give you a general overview of how it works.

STEP ONE: THE RIGHT TO BE IDENTIFIED

Under federal law, every child with a disability has the right to be identified as eligible for special education. In a public school, a parent, teacher or other school professional can make a recommendation to the school's Multi-Disciplinary Team. The team is a group of school professionals who come together to see if there is a problem, and if so, what is to be done about it. In a private school, there will also be a team of people you can call on to discuss your child's needs. Ask your child's teacher to organize a 'team meeting.'

If the team determines there's no major problems with a child's rate and level of academic progress or behavior, they might just brainstorm ideas for handling small problems. They might decide to 'wait and see' and meet again in a few months.

"Our IEP meeting was great. I'd been dreading it for months but when it happened, it was all just very businesslike. Nothing like the horror stories you read online. They had the goals and the accommodations – everything we could have hoped for. I'm starting to feel hopeful again."

RTI is a movement many school systems have adopted to increase the number of children who can get help.

Response to Intervention (RTI)

In public school, your child can access extra help without being determined eligible for special education services. RTI is a movement many school systems have adopted to increase the number of children who can get help. RTI means offering extra help to children as part of regular education. Children can get varying levels of help under RTI, such as a smaller reading group led by a reading specialist, or support from a paraeducator.

If the child still does not make progress with all the interventions that can be provided within the regular education setting (the classroom), he or she should be considered for special education.

The idea behind RTI is that no child should have to 'wait to fail' before getting assistance. Keep in mind though that RTI is not a substitute for psychological testing. Failing to make progress despite RTI does not automatically mean your child has a diagnosis.

As part of RTI, schools must conduct regular progress screenings. Note that if a child is not making an appropriate rate of progress (progressing too slowly or not at all), it is not the same as the testing needed to determine eligibility.

Importantly, just because a child is receiving extra help through RTI, it does not mean that testing should not be done. If a child is struggling, there is NO reason to go through all levels of RTI before starting the eligibility process. Parents can request the school test at any time (though the school might disagree).

Keep in mind that RTI is supposed to include structured interventions that are part of a plan for your child. RTI is supposed to be time-limited, not go on forever. Finally, the child's response to interventions must be assessed in order to determine if the interventions are having the desired effect.

If the team decides there's enough of a concern that more information is needed, the next step is to determine eligibility. This typically begins with testing. The school cannot test your child without your consent. Under the law, testing has to cover all areas of need. If you've used Part Two of this book, you are ready to describe your child's areas of need!

STEP TWO: ELIGIBILITY

Not every child who has a disability is eligible for special education services. The key to accessing special education is that the child must have a disability that has an educational impact.

The words 'educational impact' are often interpreted differently by different members of the team. Parents often see an educational impact if the child is not performing up to his or her potential. The law guarantees every student a 'free and appropriate' education, not an ideal one. The law requires that the school do what is needed to ensure that the child makes progress at the appropriate rate and level.

Educational impact is not the same as saying that the child is below grade level. Educational impact is not determined by grade level achievement alone. Certainly if his or her academics fall below grade level, the school is more likely to agree that services are warranted.

Remember that progress is about both rate and level. If you have a child who is still on grade level but whose progress has stalled, that is still an educational impact. Educational impact can also include the child's ability to 'access the curriculum.' If a child has emotional or behavior issues that significantly interfere with academics, social functioning, or relationships with teachers, he may be found eligible for services.

It may seem that the school is resistant to testing your child or starting the eligibility process. This is because schools want to have as few children receiving special education services as possible. Offering services costs the school a lot, both in funds and in staff needs. It is expensive. Schools want to have enough resources left to serve the children with the most significant disabilities. What parents see as major problems might not seem like such a big deal to the multidisciplinary team, who does this day in and day out!

If a child has emotional or behavior issues that significantly interfere with academics, social functioning, or relationships with teachers, he or she may be found eligible for services.

Others will insist on doing their own evaluations, even if you had the testing done by a world-famous psychologist.

STEP 3: DIAGNOSES AND CODES

Once the testing is done, the team re-convenes to discuss it. Some schools will let you use your own test results if the assessor is trusted. Others will insist on doing their own evaluations, even if you had the testing done by a world-famous psychologist. By law, the school has to consider private evaluation results with those obtained by school staff.

If the school did the testing, you must receive a copy and have it explained to you *before* the meeting! The last thing you want is to be caught off guard in front of a room full of professionals. Remember, a school psychologist will not generally make a diagnosis, but may say something like, "Bobby's pattern of strengths and weaknesses is consistent with ADHD." It is the team that officially determines if your child is eligible, not the psychologist.

At this point, two things are likely to happen.

1. **The team may say that the testing does not support finding your child eligible for services.** There may be a diagnosis, but the team may argue that there is no educational impact of the disability. If you disagree, the team must provide you with information about what you can do (usually they give you a booklet called *Procedural Rights and Safeguards*). Most parents fail to realize the value of this booklet. **It is absolutely crucial that you read this booklet – it describes all your rights!** At this point, you may decide to get other testing or hire an advocate. Or you may decide to pursue other options like finding a new school or hiring a tutor.

2. **The team may determine that the child is eligible for special education services.** This means that the team agrees – there is a disability that has a significant educational impact. They have two choices for how to serve the child. First, they can offer a **504 Plan**. Second, they can offer an **Individualized Education Program.**

Parents must agree to any and all special education services.

The Service Provision Code

Part of determining eligibility is selecting a Service Provision Code. The *Individuals with Disabilities Act* (IDEA) mandates that children served under special education have a code, so your child will receive a code. The code may be different from his or her diagnosis.

The 14 Codes include categories such as: learning disabilities, speech language delays, autism, visual impairments, etc.

There is no separate code for ADHD. Kids with ADHD may be coded as *Other Health Impairment* (OHI). This is the same category kids with medical problems fall into. The code is not supposed to determine placement.

THE 504 PLAN: ACCOMMODATIONS FOR YOUR CHILD

The 504 Plan is actually part of the *Americans with Disabilities Act*. It allows for the provision of reasonable accommodations if the status quo discriminates against someone with a disability. If a disability negatively impacts a 'Major Life Activity' (e.g. learning, attending school, reading, writing) then a child has the right to reasonable accommodations.

Many children with ADHD can be well served with a 504 Plan.
An IEP is not necessarily better. It depends on what your child actually needs (the test report should lay out a description of your child's needs in the Recommendations section). A 504 Plan is more desirable than informal accommodations, because you have legal recourse if the school does not make a good faith effort to honor it.

If your child is in private school, you may still have a 504 Plan or accommodations plan.
The plan may be called a Learning Support Plan (or something similar). Private schools do not have to follow the same rules that public schools do. If you have a support plan in a private school, school staff have much greater say with regards to if, or how, they will accommodate your child's needs.

A 504 Plan is a list of accommodations.
Once the list is accepted and signed by members of the multidisciplinary team, it becomes a legal document. Your child is legally entitled to the accommodations in the 504 Plan. Each school system has a list of accommodations to choose from. Remember, the school will want to give the fewest possible accommodations to help the child. This is not necessarily a bad thing, but parents often want many more than they are likely to qualify for. The decision of which accommodations to have in the Plan is the multidisciplinary team's to make. The accommodations are supposed to be selected based on what the test data shows.

If a disability negatively impacts a 'Major Life Activity' (e.g. learning, attending school, reading, writing) then a child has a right to reasonable accommodations.

Common accommodations include:

- Extended time
- Use of assistive technology
- Preferential seating
- Access to a coach/study hall class
- A behavior plan

Friction often comes from parents and schools differing on what 'reasonable' actually means.

ADA is the same law that requires public buildings to have ramps and elevators, or to allow service animals inside. A 504 Plan means that the regular education classroom will be tweaked to help reduce the impact of your child's disability on her functioning.

INDIVIDUALIZED EDUCATION PROGRAMS: DIFFERENTIATED INSTRUCTION

Being eligible for an IEP means that your child needs something more than what the regular education classroom can provide (in at least one area).

A 504 Plan allows for reasonable accommodations in the regular education setting. **An Individualized Education Program (IEP) means that the child's needs cannot be met without differentiated instruction.** IEP provisions come from the federal *Individuals with Disabilities Act* (IDEA). Being eligible for an IEP means that your child needs something more than what the regular education classroom can provide (in at least one area). The IEP guarantees that your child will receive an *individualized* education program designed to address all of your child's areas of need.

An IEP is a long, complicated legal document. The basic components of the IEP include:

- Service Code
- Educational Placement in the least restrictive environment
- Supplementary Aids and Services (what interventions your child will receive)*
- Related Services (therapies)**
- Goals and Objectives
- Behavior Intervention Plan (BIP)
- Accommodations (just like the 504 Plan)
- Transition Plan (for children over 13)
- Extended School Year (ESY) determination (for special education summer school)

* *Supplementary Aids and Services* refers to the meat of what 'special education' will be provided. This covers things like special classes, time with the reading specialist, assistive technology.

** *Related Services* refers to therapies provided by Speech Language Pathologists, Occupational Therapists, Physical Therapists and Psychologists. In order to access each kind of professional service, you'll need a separate evaluation and eligibility determination.

THE BEHAVIOR INTERVENTION PLAN: PART OF THE IEP

A BIP is needed if your child's unwanted behavior persists despite the regular classroom behavior system.

The Behavior Intervention Plan is often an area schools don't do as well. The BIP should be created using a Functional Behavior Analysis (FBA – a formal, structured observation for data gathering). A special educator or school psychologist typically conducts the FBA and writes the BIP. The BIP may also be based on psychological test data as well.

Behavior systems in most classrooms work great – for the kids who really don't need them! As Dr. Ross Greene points out, the same kids are the ones always getting the rewards. Of course the converse is true, the kids who really need to learn new skills are the same ones who rarely get the rewards (and are most likely to always be on 'level red' or the equivalent). Most of the generic behavior plans are not very effective for kids who have skill deficits (the kids who are struggling to meet behavioral expectations). When psychologists talk about skill deficits, we are not referring to academic skills. Academic skill deficits are easier to fix. Children with ADHD are immature in their acquisition of 'soft' skills, such as being able to exert self-control, tolerate frustration or self-motivate.

In the previous sections, I covered why kids with ADHD struggle with self-control, hyperactivity, and motivation problems. Remember that our kids with ADHD also may not have the 'soft' skills they need to cope with the demands of the classroom. For example, they might not be able to 'talk themselves down' when they become frustrated.

The BIP should be oriented around increasing 'positive opposite' behaviors.

Positive opposite behaviors (a coin termed by Dr. Alan Kazdin) are desirable or tolerable behaviors that replace undesirable ones. A positive opposite behavior is using a quiet voice instead of shouting, or handling a fidget instead of tapping a pencil during seatwork. Remember, discipline is about teaching, not punishing.

The BIP should offer the child frequent positive feedback about what he's doing right.

It also needs to have a plan for giving almost immediate feedback when an undesirable behavior appears. Most plans make the mistake of letting kids know how they have done hours after the undesirable behavior occurred – no child remembers much about what happened hours ago, much less about what events led up to it! Our kids with ADHD are even more 'in the moment' than their peers. Positive and negative feedback needs to be delivered as soon as possible!

Remember that our kids with ADHD also may not have the 'soft' skills they need to cope with the demands of the classroom. For example, they might not be able to 'talk themselves down' when they become frustrated.

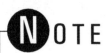

Dr. Alan Kazdin makes an excellent point about negative consequences – small ones work best! Taking one or two points away is more effective than a large punishment like having to stay home from a field trip or missing the class Halloween party. Points work well because the teacher can give them liberally. The child should be focused on earning lots and lots of points that are tied to small rewards and privileges. Small rewards work even better than big ones.

A BIP is usually oriented around a point or token system.

Marbles or puff balls in a jar work very well for younger children, especially if they can put the objects in the jar themselves. Some children like to have a chart that they can color in when they earn a reward. It is critical to start out 'setting the bar' very low so the child is guaranteed an introductory period of success. In the early stages, reward often and give lots of positive feedback so the child knows exactly why she earned the point. Once they buy in and start earning rewards, they are on a good trajectory to keep improving.

What to look for in a good BIP:

- Addresses antecedents/triggers and trouble spots
- Offers rewards for 'positive opposite' behaviors
- Sets the bar low at first, then raises it gradually to build success
- Is easy for a teacher to use
- Allows for immediate positive reinforcement
- Allows for immediate redirection or removal of 1-2 points for transgressions
- Allows the child to earn back points if he changes his behavior or makes amends
- Has a reinforcement system that is visible to the child
- Is appealing to the child
- Points are tied to small rewards or privileges
- The child has input into what rewards and privileges he wishes to work for
- The child never loses recess, PE or other specials unless his behavior makes it unsafe for him to participate
- Avoids suspension (which has not been shown to be effective)

ADVOCATES AND ATTORNEYS _____

**If you are not getting what you need from special education,
there are professionals who can help.**
Within the school system, you may get some help from parent advocates,
pupil personal workers, or mediators. However, these professionals work for
the school. Their job is to help you and the school come to a solution that is
acceptable to the school system.

ADVOCATES

**An advocate is someone you hire *outside the school system*
who is well trained in special education law and policy.**
Good advocates have excellent experience in special education, and can offer
constructive suggestions to get a team 'un-stuck.' They are skilled negotiators
who foster collaboration.

Remember, *anyone can call him or herself an advocate.*
Avoid advocates whose main qualification is that they've 'been through this
themselves.' They may have the best intentions, but unless they have formal
training, they may not know enough about law and policy to be effective
advocates. I have seen advocates who actually made the situation worse for their
clients because they did not know what they were doing.

**Your best bet for an advocate is someone who has
worked in special education.**
Preferably as a teacher, administrator, or school psychologist. These professionals
have the appropriate training and credentials to give you trustworthy advice.

**Also beware of advocates who 'become part of the family'
or who try to provide you with therapy or amateur counseling.**
Your advocate is not your buddy or your counselor. Your advocate should not be
coming to dinner at your house. Your advocate should not be playing therapist
with your child. A good advocate needs to maintain professional boundaries so
he or she can be objective when giving you advice! A good advocate must be
ready to tell you things you might not want to hear. Your advocate is going to
be on your side, but as with any advisor, should maintain enough professional
distance to remain objective.

Select an advocate who focuses on collaboration.
Avoid the advocate who immediately takes an aggressive 'us versus them' stance.
While you want the advocate to be on your side, someone who makes everybody
angry will just make your child's situation worse. Avoid the advocate to tries
to 'win' by making threats or trying to show why she's the smartest person in
the room. Even if she's right, the rest of the team will not give an inch to please
someone like that! Never hire an advocate who is personally abrasive.

A good advocate must be ready to tell you things you might not want to hear. Your advocate is going to be on your side, but as with any advisor, should maintain enough professional distance to remain objective.

While you want someone who will fight for you, your ideal outcome is to prevail without having to go to court.

SPECIAL EDUCATION ATTORNEYS

The most important qualities in a special education attorney are expertise and ethics.

Your attorney should be honest with you about the best path to take, even if that path is not the most lucrative for him.
Your attorney should also be willing to tell you if she does not think your request is in your child's best interest.

Attorneys vary in terms of how collaborative they like to be.
Some function more like high-powered advocates, others specialize in litigation. Your attorney should focus on avoiding due process (going to court/litigation) unless it is truly necessary. Going to court is very expensive and terribly stressful. While you want someone who will fight for you, your ideal outcome is to prevail without having to go to court.

CHAPTER FOURTEEN:

CREATING YOUR 12-MONTH ACTION PLAN

Each year, it is a good idea to create a formal Action Plan. This regular 12-month review helps you stay on top of what's working, where new opportunities have emerged, and therapies and interventions that may no longer be needed.

Dates covered by this plan: _____

My child's age during this plan: _____

What are the goals I have in setting this plan?
List any specific behaviors or concerns that you want addressed during the course of the coming year. Think about immediate concerns and also look ahead at the calendar: what upcoming events might pose challenges for your child academically, socially, and in the family?

_____

_____

_____

_____

_____

_____

_____

_____

_____

_____

_____

_____

IN EACH AREA BELOW, WHAT SPECIFIC STEPS DO YOU WANT TO TAKE?

Disclosure.
Goals might include developing an elevator pitch, listing who you should inform about your child's ADHD and how/when you are going to tell them.

_____

_____

_____

_____

Testing.
Goals might include deciding how satisfied you are with how (and who) made your child's ADHD diagnosis. If you want to consider new testing, goals might include finding the right resource (school or private) to do the testing, and establishing the timeline on which the testing will be completed.

_____

_____

_____

_____

Lifestyle Changes.
What lifestyle changes can you make for your child? How will you achieve the goals of increasing exercise, improving sleep, or reducing junk food? What changes will you make in family routine or other areas? And what about _YOU_ – what changes are needed to give you the space and time for 'self-care' that is necessary to support your child and your family?

_____

_____

_____

_____

Medication.

Are you going to pursue medication? If so, what type of a physician will you consult? What specific questions will you want answered? What steps do you need to take to explore what portion of the costs will be covered by insurance?

_____

_____

_____

_____

_____

Therapy/Skills Training.

Are you going to find a therapist for your child? If yes, will you look for individual or group therapy? What 'homework' can you do to prepare for your initial consultation with the provider (e.g. do you need to gather information on the diagnosis, summarize your concerns, etc.).

_____

_____

_____

_____

_____

Educational Interventions.

Will you seek special education services for your child? What services do you think would be most helpful? How will you learn about the process your school uses for assessing and awarding accommodations/special education resources? Would it help you to have an advocate during this process? If so, what type of support would you like and who can refer you to the professional help you need?

_____

_____

_____

_____

_____

ABOUT THE AUTHOR

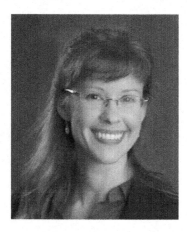

DR. REBECCA RESNIK

Dr. Rebecca Resnik is a licensed psychologist and founding partner of Rebecca Resnik and Associates, specialists in psychological care and testing.

Dr. Resnik has earned a Doctor of Psychology from The George Washington University. She also holds a Master of Education in Special Education from The University of Maryland at College Park, as well as a Bachelor of Science, Special Education (Cum Laude). Dr. Resnik completed her psychology internship training in Pediatric Psychology and Neuropsychology at Mount Washington Pediatric Hospital. Her postdoctoral residency in Psychological Assessment was completed at MindWell Psychology in Virginia. Dr. Resnik is a Licensed Psychologist in the state of Maryland.

She has served as a voting member of the Maryland Psychological Association's (MPA) Board of Directors, Maryland Psychological Association since 2011, and has been recognized for leadership in her service to MPA. Dr. Resnik is also a member of the GTLD Network, Exceptional Minds (X-Minds), Learning Disabilities Association of Montgomery County, and Women Business Owners of Montgomery County. Her research interests include applications of computational linguistics in psychology. She was co-organizer of the first Computational Linguistics and Clinical Psychology workshop held at the Association for Computational Linguistics' Annual International Conference, and continues to be a reviewer for the Workshop.

Dr. Resnik enjoys sharing her love of psychology. She serves as a medical expert for MedHelp for the ADHD and Learning Disability forums. She has appeared on *Fox News, Let's Talk Live,* and *Voice of America*. Dr. Resnik regularly contributes to articles about psychology and child development. She loves giving parent education talks, professional training/continuing education for psychologists, and conducting teacher training for private schools.

Dr. Resnik is married to a college professor and resides in Bethesda, MD. She and her husband love raising their two rambunctious young boys. Her stepson is a recent graduate of Brown University, who is currently working as a political consultant in Washington DC.

RESOURCES AND REFERENCES

RESOURCES

The Energetic Brain by Dr. Cecil Reynolds

The Kazdin Method for Parenting the Disruptive Child by Dr. Alan Kazdin

Driven to Distraction by Dr. Edward Hallowell and Dr. John Ratey, also the website sparkinglife.org

Understanding Girls with ADHD, Updated and Revised: How They Feel and Why They Do What They Do by Dr. Kathleen Nadeau

Smart but Scattered by Dr. Peg Dawson

Center for Parent Education and Resources, a public resource provided by the government to help parents understand special education law and policy http://www.parentcenterhub.org/

How to Talk So Kids Will Listen & Listen So Kids Will Talk by Adele Faber and Elaine Mazlish (also *How to Talk So Kids Can Learn* and *How to Talk So Teens Will Listen*)

Lives in the Balance (livesinthebalance.org), Dr. Ross Green's *Collaborative Problem-Solving Approach*. For teachers, *Lost at School* by Dr. Ross Green. See also *The Explosive Child*

Smart Kids with Learning Difficulties, Overcoming Obstacles and Realizing Potential by Rich Weinfeld

The Special Needs Advocacy Resource Book by Rich Weinfeld

Hunter and His Amazing Remote Control: A Fun Hands-on Way to Teach Self-Control to ADHD Children by Lori Ann Copeland

FOR CHILDREN:

Learning to Feel Good and Stay Cool by Dr. Judith Glasser

Learning to Be Kind and Understand Differences: Empathy Skills for Kids with AD/HD by Dr. Judith Glasser

The Survival Guide for Kids with ADHD by Dr. John Taylor

REFERENCES

Barkley, R.A. (2014). *Attention-Deficit Hyperactivity Disorder: A Handbook for Diagnosis and Treatment*. Guilford Publications. Retrieved from https://books.google.com/books?hl=en&lr=&id=0J0gBQAAQBAJ&pgis=1

Barkley, R. A. (2000). *Taking Charge of ADHD: The Complete, Authoritative Guide for Parents*. Guilford Press. Retrieved from https://books.google.com/books?id=-HOzQgAACAAJ&pgis=1

Beljan, P., Bree, K. D., Reuter, A. E. F., Reuter, S. D., & Wingers, L. (2014). Private Pediatric Neuropsychology Practice Multimodal Treatment of ADHD: An Applied Approach. *Applied Neuropsychology: Child*, 3(July), 188–196. doi:10.1080/21622965.2013.875300

BRIEF (Behavior Rating Inventory of Executive Function). (n.d.). Retrieved November 10, 2015, from http://www4.parinc.com/Products/Product.aspx?ProductID=BRIEF

Carmichael, J. A., Kubas, H. A., Carlson, H. L., Fitzer, K. R., Wilcox, G., Lemay, J.-F., ... Hale, J. B. (2015). Reconsidering "inattention" in attention-deficit hyperactivity disorder: implications for neuropsychological assessment and intervention. *Applied Neuropsychology. Child*, 4(2), 97–105. doi:10.1080/21622965.2015.1005481

CEFI - Comprehensive Executive Function Inventory. (n.d.). Retrieved November 10, 2015, from http://www.mhs.com/product.aspx?gr=cli&id=overview&prod=cefi

Center for Parent Information and Resources. (n.d.). Retrieved November 10, 2015, from http://www.parentcenterhub.org/

Conners CBRS - Conners Comprehensive Behavior Rating Scales. (n.d.). Retrieved November 10, 2015, from http://www.mhs.com/product.aspx?gr=edu&id=overview&prod=cbrs

Dawson, P., & Guare, R. (2011). *Smart but Scattered: The Revolutionary "Executive Skills" Approach to Helping Kids Reach Their Potential* (Vol. 30). Guilford Press. Retrieved from https://books.google.com/books?id=J5MA8e5YHmQC&pgis=1

Duckworth, A. L., Peterson, C., Matthews, M. D., & Kelly, D. R. (n.d.). Grit: Perseverance and passion for long-term goals. Journal of Personality and Social Psychology, Vol 92(6), Jun 2007, 1087-1101

Duff, C. T., & Sulla, E. M. (2015). Measuring Executive Function in the Differential Diagnosis of Attention-Deficit/Hyperactivity Disorder: Does It Really Tell Us Anything? *Applied Neuropsychology. Child*, 4(3), 188–96. doi:10.1080/216229 65.2013.848329

Emotional Disorders: A Neuropsychological, Psychopharmacological, and Educational Perspective. (2010). School Neuropsych Press. Retrieved from https://books.google.com/books?id=aLRZAAAAYAAJ&pgis=1

Faber, A., & Mazlish, E. (2012). *How to Talk So Kids Will Listen & Listen So Kids Will Talk.* Simon and Schuster. Retrieved from https://books.google.com/books?hl=en&lr=&id=LG69eA4wvKoC&pgis=1

Faber, A., Mazlish, E., & Faber, J. (2012). *How to Talk So Kids Will Listen & Listen So Kids Will Talk.* Simon and Schuster. Retrieved from https://books.google.com/books?id=bSJdeLSEQ-IC&pgis=1

Feifer, S. G., & Fina, P. A. De. (2000). *The Neuropsychology of Reading Disorders: Diagnosis and Intervention Workbook.* School Neuropsych Press, LLC. Retrieved from https://books.google.com/books?id=jHIXPQAACAAJ&pgis=1

Feifer, S. G., & Fina, P. A. De. (2002). *The Neuropsychology of Written Language Disorders: Diagnosis and Intervention.* School Neuropsych Press. Retrieved from https://books.google.com/books?id=KKjSAAAACAAJ&pgis=1

Ginnot, H. (1973). Between parent and child. Retrieved from https://scholar.google.com/scholar?cluster=12446337544392294247&hl=en&as_sdt=20000005&sciodt=0,21#0

Gioia, G. a, Isquith, P. K., Guy, S. C., & Kenworthy, L. (2000). Behavior rating inventory of executive function. *Child Neuropsychology: A Journal on Normal and Abnormal Development in Childhood and Adolescence*, 6(3), 235–238. doi:10.1076/chin.6.3.235.3152

Gottman, J. M. (1999). *The Marriage Clinic: A Scientifically-based Marital Therapy.* W.W. Norton. Retrieved from https://books.google.com/books?hl=en&lr=&id=cQsX_UgESWUC&pgis=1

Graham, S., & Harris, K. R. (2005). *Writing Better: Effective Strategies for Teaching Students with Learning Difficulties.* Paul H. Brookes Publishing Company. Retrieved from https://books.google.com/books?id=QS90QgAACAAJ&pgis=1

Graham, S., & Mason, L. H. (2008). *Powerful Writing Strategies for All Students.* Paul H. Brookes Publishing Company. Retrieved from https://books.google.com/books?id=15coAQAAMAAJ&pgis=1

Greene, R. W. (2014). *Lost at School: Why Our Kids with Behavioral Challenges Are Falling Through the Cracks and How We Can Help Them.* Simon and Schuster. Retrieved from https://books.google.com/books?id=LQaZBAAAQBAJ&pgis=1

Greene, R. W., & PhD. (2014). *The Explosive Child: A New Approach for Understanding and Parenting Easily Frustrated, Chronically Inflexible Children.* HarperCollins. Retrieved from https://books.google.com/books?id=HHIpAgAAQBAJ&pgis=1

Guare, R. (2014). Context in the development of executive functions in children. *Applied Neuropsychology. Child*, 3(3), 226–32. doi:10.1080/21622965.2013.870015

Hale, J. B., Alfonso, V. C., Berninger, V., Bracken, B., Christo, C., Clark, E., … Goldstein, S. (2010). Critical Issues in Response-to-Intervention, Comprehensive Evaluation, and Specific Learning Disabilities Identification and Intervention: An Expert White Paper Consensus. *Learning Disability Quarterly*, 33(3), 223–236. doi:Article

Hale, J. B., & Fiorello, C. A. (2004). *School Neuropsychology: A Practitioner's Handbook.* Guilford Press. Retrieved from https://books.google.com/books?id=A6No2zeGePkC&pgis=1

Hale, J. B., & Fitzer, K. R. (2015). Evaluating orbital-ventral medial system regulation of personal attention: a critical need for neuropsychological assessment and intervention. *Applied Neuropsychology. Child*, 4(2), 106–15. doi:10.1080/21622965.2015.1005486

Hale, J. B., Reddy, L. a, Decker, S. L., Thompson, R., Henzel, J., Teodori, A., … Denckla, M. B. (2009). Development and validation of an attention-deficit/hyperactivity disorder (ADHD) executive function and behavior rating screening battery. *Journal of Clinical and Experimental Neuropsychology*, 31(8), 897–912. doi:10.1080/13803390802687423

Hale, J. B., Reddy, L. a, Semrud-Clikeman, M., Hain, L. a, Whitaker, J., Morley, J., … Jones, N. (2011). Executive impairment determines ADHD medication response: implications for academic achievement. *Journal of Learning Disabilities*, 44(2), 196–212. doi:10.1177/0022219410391191

Hallowell, E. M. M., & Ratey, J. J. (2011). *Driven to Distraction: Recognizing and Coping with Attention Deficit Disorder from Childhood Through Adulthood.* Anchor Books. Retrieved from https://books.google.com/books?id=uPBoFwCJtEYC&pgis=1

Handbook of Neurodevelopmental and Genetic Disorders in Children, 2/e.
(2010). Guilford Press. Retrieved from https://books.google.com/
books?id=sGPHyIMVOMgC&pgis=1

Isquith, P. K., Roth, R. M., Kenworthy, L., & Gioia, G. (2014). Contribution of Rating
Scales to Intervention for Executive Dysfunction. *Applied Neuropsychology.*
Child, (April 2014), 37–41. doi:10.1080/21622965.2013.870014

Jobes, D. A. (2006). *Managing Suicidal Risk: A Collaborative Approach.*
Guilford Press. Retrieved from https://books.google.com/
books?id=UgOWO8IUqbIC&pgis=1

Joyce, A., & Hrin, S. (2015). Attention: an evolving construct. *Applied*
Neuropsychology. Child, 4(2), 80–8. doi:10.1080/21622965.2015.1005476

Kahneman, D. (2011). *Thinking, Fast and Slow.* Farrar, Straus and Giroux.
Retrieved from https://books.google.com/books?id=ZuKTvERuPG8C&pgis=1

Kazdin, A. E. (2005). *Parent Management Training: Treatment for Oppositional,*
Aggressive, and Antisocial Behavior in Children and Adolescents.
Oxford University Press. Retrieved from https://books.google.com/
books?hl=en&lr=&id=FdQPdCo5OA8C&pgis=1

Kazdin, A. E., & Rotella, C. (2009). *The Kazdin Method for Parenting the Defiant*
Child: With No Pills, No Therapy, No Contest of Wills. Houghton Mifflin.
Retrieved from https://books.google.com/books?id=wtTmoiQ0GRQC&pgis=1

Koziol, L. F., Barker, L. A., & Jansons, L. (2015). Attention and other constructs:
evolution or revolution? *Applied Neuropsychology. Child*, 4(2), 123–31. doi:10
.1080/21622965.2015.1005482

Koziol, L. F., Joyce, A. W., & Wurglitz, G. (2014). The neuropsychology of attention:
revisiting the "Mirsky model." *Applied Neuropsychology. Child*, 3(4), 297–307.
doi:10.1080/21622965.2013.870016

Lezak, M. D., Howieson, D. B., Bigler, E. D., & Tranel, D. (2012).
Neuropsychological Assessment. Oxford University Press. Retrieved from
https://books.google.com/books?id=hryvBAAAQBAJ&pgis=1

Lives in the Balance and Dr. Greene's approach. (n.d.). Retrieved November 10,
2015, from http://livesinthebalance.org/

McCloskey, G., Perkins, L. A., & Diviner, B. Van. (2008). *Assessment and*
Intervention for Executive Function Difficulties. Taylor & Francis. Retrieved
from https://books.google.com/books?id=J06TAgAAQBAJ&pgis=1

MD, D. J. S. (2014). *Brainstorm: The Power and Purpose of the Teenage Brain.* Penguin Publishing Group. Retrieved from https://books.google.com/books?id=SOi4yca7FSsC&pgis=1

Nadeau, K. G., Littman, E., & Quinn, P. O. (1999). *Understanding girls with attention deficit hyperactivity disorder* (Vol. 1). Advantage Books. Retrieved from https://books.google.com/books?id=rpLgAAAAMAAJ&pgis=1

Organization, W. H. (2004). *International Statistical Classification of Diseases and Related Health Problems, Volume 1.* World Health Organization. Retrieved from https://books.google.com/books?id=Tw5eAtsatiUC&pgis=1

Otero, T. M., Barker, L. A., & Naglieri, J. A. (2014). Executive function treatment and intervention in schools. *Applied Neuropsychology. Child*, 3(3), 205–14. doi:10.1080/21622965.2014.897903

Pessoa, L. (2013). *The Cognitive-Emotional Brain: From Interactions to Integration.* MIT Press. Retrieved from https://books.google.com/books?id=JTsEAQAAQBAJ&pgis=1

Pinker, S. (2003). *How the Mind Works.* Penguin Books Limited. Retrieved from https://books.google.com/books?id=xhIgYdSq64gC&pgis=1

Ratey, J. J., & Hagerman, E. (2008). *Spark: The Revolutionary New Science of Exercise and the Brain.* Little, Brown. Retrieved from https://books.google.com/books?hl=en&lr=&id=zM_9Ft1j40UC&pgis=1

Reynolds, C. R., Vannest, K. J., & Harrison, J. R. (2011). *The Energetic Brain: Understanding and Managing ADHD.* John Wiley & Sons. Retrieved from https://books.google.com/books?id=sT1M9B_pgCkC&pgis=1

Rosenberg, L. (2015). The Associations Between Executive Functions' Capacities, Performance Process Skills, and Dimensions of Participation in Activities of Daily Life Among Children of Elementary School Age. *Applied Neuropsychology. Child*, 4(3), 148–56. doi:10.1080/21622965.2013.821652

Shaywitz, S., & M.D. (2008). *Overcoming Dyslexia: A New and Complete Science-Based Program for Reading Problems at Any Level.* Knopf Doubleday Publishing Group. Retrieved from https://books.google.com/books?id=jHU02hSTCJsC&pgis=1

Silver, L. B., & M.D. (2010). *Dr. Larry Silver's Advice to Parents on ADHD: Second Edition.* Crown Publishing Group. Retrieved from https://books.google.com/books?id=djLYnmOfY_sC&pgis=1

Sparking Life: Optimize your brain function with exercise! (n.d.). Retrieved November 10, 2015, from http://www.sparkinglife.org/

Statistics, A. P. A. T. F. on N. and. (1980). *Diagnostic and Statistical Manual of Mental Disorders.* American Psychiatric Association. Retrieved from https://books.google.com/books?id=NsnKnQEACAAJ&pgis=1

Townsend, B. L. (2000). The Disproportionate Discipline of African American Learners: Reducing School Suspensions and Expulsions. *Exceptional Children*, 66(3), 381–391. doi:10.1177/001440290006600308

Transforming Diagnosis. (n.d.). Retrieved from http://www.nimh.nih.gov/about/director/2013/transforming-diagnosis.shtml

Wasserman, T., & Wasserman, L. D. (2015). The misnomer of attention-deficit hyperactivity disorder. *Applied Neuropsychology. Child*, 4(2), 116–22. doi:10.1080/21622965.2015.1005487

Wechsler Intelligence Scale for Children®-Fifth Edition. (n.d.). Retrieved November 10, 2015, from http://www.pearsonclinical.com/psychology/products/100000771/wechsler-intelligence-scale-for-childrensupsupfifth-edition--wisc-v.html

Weinfeld, R. (2006). *Smart Kids with Learning Difficulties: Overcoming Obstacles and Realizing Potential.* Prufrock Press Inc. Retrieved from https://books.google.com/books?id=68ZkHgndd8UC&pgis=1

Weinfeld, R., & Davis, M. (2008). *Special Needs Advocacy Resource Book: What You Can Do Now to Advocate for Your Exceptional Child's Education.* Prufrock Press Inc. Retrieved from https://books.google.com/books?id=tOdTGHi5w-4C&pgis=1

Wolraich, M. L. (1995). The Effect of Sugar on Behavior or Cognition in Children. *JAMA*, 274(20), 1617. doi:10.1001/jama.1995.03530200053037

INDEX

(continued)

(continued)

Made in the USA
Middletown, DE
12 December 2019